Computed
Tomography

PAULA COLE.

Computed Tomography

STEWART C. BUSHONG, Sc.D., F.A.C.R., F.A.C.M.P.

Professor of Radiologic Science
Department of Radiology
Baylor College of Medicine
Houston, Texas

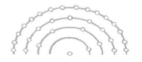

ESSENTIALS OF MEDICAL IMAGING SERIES

McGraw-Hill

Health Professions Division

New York   St. Louis   San Francisco   Auckland   Bogotá   Caracas   Lisbon   London   Madrid
Mexico City   Milan   Montreal   New Delhi   San Juan
Singapore   Sydney   Tokyo   Toronto

McGraw-Hill

A Division of The **McGraw·Hill** *Companies*

Computed Tomography

Essentials of Medical Imaging Series

Copyright © 2000 by The **McGraw-Hill Companies**, Inc. All rights reserved.
Printed in the United States of America. Except as permitted under the
United States Copyright Act of 1976, no part of this publication may be
reproduced or distributed in any form or by any means, or stored in a data
base or retrieval system without the prior written permission of the publisher.

8 9 0   CUS CUS   10

ISBN 0-07-134354-7

This book was set in Berkeley by V&M Graphics.
The editors were John J. Dolan, Sally Barhydt, and Barbara Holton.
The production supervisor was Rohnda Barnes.
The text designer was Jose R. Fonfrias.
The cover designer was Robert Freese.
Phoenix Book Technoligies was printer and binder.

This book is printed on acid-free paper.

Cataloging-in-Publication data is on file for this title at the Library of Congress.

Dedicated to

Sharon Glaze and Benjamin Archer

my friends and colleagues for many years. Their continuing effort, commitment and support has allowed me the time to write books like this. Thanks.

Contents

Preface

IMAGING SCIENCE has changed considerably over the past twenty years. These changes have brought an incredible increase in information, understanding and innovation. One result is that, today, imaging technologists, medical physicists and radiologists must know far more than their predecessors. The fund of knowledge required of these imaging professionals, especially the imaging technologist, for any of the professional examinations is so vast that the demands on learning and teaching are considerable.

Accompanying this expansion of knowledge are substantial changes in occupational opportunities. Limited credentialing, cross-training and job splitting are changing the required competence and responsibilities of those involved in medical imaging. The principal focus of these changes is to obtain more production with fewer professionals. Managed healthcare will continue to exert economic and occupational restrictions on the imaging professional.

This book is one in a series designed to make the learning process easier for the imaging professional. Computed tomography was predicted by many in the early 1980s to die a slow death because of the introduction of magnetic resonance imaging. However, with the introduction of spiral CT in 1990 and multislice spiral CT in 1992, computed tomography clinical applications are rapidly increasing. It is now possible to image the entire body in a single breathhold. This volume presents the essential facts of the physics of computed tomography.

Additional volumes in this series concentrate on other specialty topics and areas of examination.

None of these volumes is a textbook. Sometimes, especially when preparing for an examination, it is easier to commit statements of fact to memory, while working with other sources to gain a better understanding of those facts. Each of these volumes contain extensive statements of fact that the author believes are essential for satisfactory completion of the respective professional examination. These volumes are well illustrated because, "A picture is work a thousand words". Where graphs, charts or tables are included, they are also accompanied with brief statements of fact. At the end of each chapter, there are practice questions patterned after the respective professional examinations, such as the ABR, ABMP, ARDMS, CNMT and especially the ARRT and its subspecialty examinations in quality management, mammography, computed tomography, cardiovascular-interventional technology and magnetic resonance imaging.

Most examination panels, especially the ARRT, principally use Type A questions: a statement or stem followed by four distractors and one correct answer. Type K questions are used less frequently. These contain multiple statements and the candidate selects the correct combination of answers. The practice question provided here are of both types.

At the end of this of this volume, there are three appendices that the student and educator will find particularly helpful. Appendix A is a rather complete glossary of terms employed in imaging science and technology. The student should pay particular attention to this appendix and attempt to know and understand each definition. You will find this very helpful at examination time. Appendix B lists the latest textbooks and additional sources of education material covering the respective information areas of this volume. Here, the student will find literature references to aid in understating through additional reading of a particular subject. The educator will find this section helpful when assigning special topics or special projects to students. Appendix C contains the answers to the practice questions.

I am particularly grateful to Yvonne Young and Robert Lapsley. Yvonne was exceptionally helpful with manuscript preparation, not only processing but also editing. Lapsley drew all of the illustrations and was very creative.

Medical imaging as practiced today in all of its forms is based on special principles of physics. To many students, physics is the most feared of subjects—it does not have to be. The purpose of this volume is to ease the learning process, prepare the student for examination and help to **MAKE PHYSICS FUN**.

STEWART C. BUSHONG

Computed Tomography

Historical Perspective

- Computed tomography (CT) has also been identified as computerized axial tomography (CAT), computerized transaxial tomography (CTAT), and digital axial tomography (DAT).

- Computed tomography results in a digital image.

- Computed tomography results in a transverse (transaxial) image.

- The principal advantage of CT imaging over other x-ray imaging is improved contrast resolution.

- Tomography is from the Greek "tomos," meaning section.

- Unfortunately, we identify an image section as a "slice." What do you suppose patients think?

- Alan Cormack originally applied reconstruction techniques in nuclear medicine. His publications on that application are dated 1964, 10 years before CT.

- Emission CT involves nuclear medicine and γ-ray emission from a patient administered a radionuclide.

- Computed tomography utilizes x-ray transmission through a patient.

a brief history of CT
- 1895 Roentgen discovers x-rays
- 1917 Radon develops reconstruction mathmatics
- 1963 Cormack formulates x-ray absorption in tissue
- 1972 Hounsfield demonstrates CT
- 1975 first whole body CT
- 1979 Hounsfield and Cormack receive Nobel Prize
- 1983 EBCT demonstrated
- 1989 spiral CT demonstrated
- 1991 multislice CT introduced

limitations of CT:
- spatial resolution
- relatively high patient dose
- z-axis reformation
- distinct artifacts

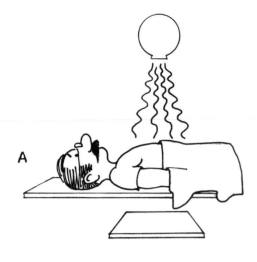

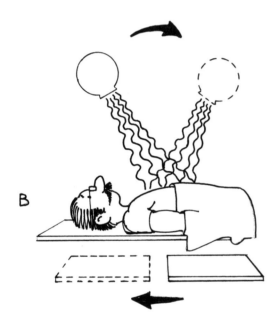

Equipment arrangement for obtaining a conventional radiograph, A, and a conventional tomograph, B.

CONVENTIONAL TOMOGRAPHY

- Conventional tomography is a radiograph obtained with a moving source image receptor assembly.

- Conventional tomography results in an image of superimposed tissues.

- There is no superimposition of tissues in CT.

- Scatter radiation reduces radiographic contrast resolution.

- Conventional tomography improves contrast resolution by blurring tissues above and below the focal plane.

- Conventional tomography does not improve spatial resolution.

- Conventional tomography results in an axial image—coronal or sagittal.

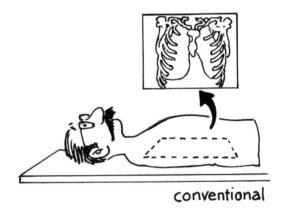

conventional

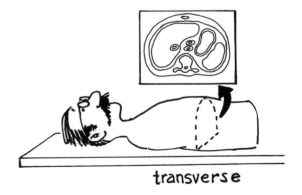

transverse

DISCOVERY

- The development of CT required the emergence of the digital computer and special mathematics.

- Godfrey Hounsfield, an engineer, and Alan Cormack, a medical physicist, shared the 1979 Nobel Prize in medicine for the development of CT.

- Cormack, a South African transplanted to Tufts University, developed the mathematics of image reconstruction by **back projection** in the 1950s and 1960s.

- Hounsfield demonstrated the first CT scanner in 1972, using Cormack's mathematics.

- Houndsfield's original attempt at CT used a gamma source—output too low, source too large.

PRINCIPLES OF OPERATION

- Hounsfield's original approach was to **translate** an object through a collimated x-ray beam and detect an image **projection**.

- The projection is a digital rendering of x-ray attenuation through the object.

- Multiple projections are obtained by **rotating** the object between translations.

- A computer-generated matrix of a section of the object is produced by back projection reconstruction—a special application of simultaneous equations.

advantages of CT over conventional radiography/tomography :
- better contrast resolution
- no superimposition of tissue
- less scatter radiation
- 3D imaging
- bone mineral assay

Chapter 1 Practice Questions

1. Computed tomography (CT) results in a/an
   a. analog image.
   b. linear image.
   c. digital image.
   d. curvilinear image.
   e. image in time.

2. Which of the following scientists were instrumental in the initial development of CT?

   1. Alan Cormack
   2. Raymond Damadian
   3. Geodfrey Hounsfield
   4. Paul Lauterbur

   a. Only 1, 2, and 3 are correct.
   b. Only 1 and 3 are correct.
   c. Only 2 and 4 are correct.
   d. Only 4 is correct.
   e. All are correct.

3. The principal advantage of CT over projection radiography is

   a. speed of image acquisition.
   b. energy resolution.
   c. contrast resolution.
   d. spatial resolution.
   e. temporal resolution.

4. Which of the following terms does not fit?

   a. section
   b. slice
   c. tomos
   d. axial
   e. volume

5. Computed tomography is otherwise identified as

   a. emission tomography.
   b. transmission tomography.
   c. reflection tomography.
   d. temporal tomography.
   e. volumetric tomography.

6. When compared to projection radiography, conventional tomography shows

   a. better spatial resolution.
   b. improved contrast resolution.
   c. reduced patient dose.
   d. relaxed quality control.
   e. less operator involvement.

7. Which of the following involves emission of a signal from a patient?

   a. CT
   b. diagnostic ultrasound
   c. magnetic resonance imaging
   d. projection radiography
   e. spiral CT

8. The data acquisition in CT results in a/an

   a. oblique image.
   b. transverse image.
   c. sagittal image.
   d. coronal image.
   e. volume image.

9. Which of the following scientists received the Nobel Prize for their work leading to CT?

    1. Alan Cormack
    2. Raymond Damadian
    3. Geodfrey Hounsfield
    4. Paul Lauterbur

    a. Only 1, 2, and 3 are correct.
    b. Only 1 and 3 are correct.
    c. Only 2 and 4 are correct.
    d. Only 4 is correct.
    e. All are correct.

10. Which of the following are characteristic limitations of CT?

    1. spatial resolution
    2. artifact generation
    3. z-axis resolution
    4. patient dose

    a. Only 1, 2, and 3 are correct.
    b. Only 1 and 3 are correct.
    c. Only 2 and 4 are correct.
    d. Only 4 is correct.
    e. All are correct.

11. A characteristic feature of a projection radiograph is

    a. poor spatial resolution.
    b. lengthy data acquisition.
    c. difficult quality control requirements.
    d. tissue superimposition.
    e. excessive patient dose.

12. Which of the following finds application in bone mineral assay for evaluation of osteoporosis?

    a. radioisotope emission tomography
    b. conventional tomography
    c. CT
    d. projection radiography
    e. fluoroscopy

13. Which of the following involves emission of a signal from a patient?

    a. CT
    b. diagnostic ultrasound
    c. projection radiography
    d. radioisotope imaging
    e. spiral CT

14. Compared to projection radiography, conventional tomography results in improved contrast resolution because

    a. imaging time is reduced.
    b. out of plane tissues are blurred.
    c. tissues are superimposed.
    d. precise beam collimation is employed.
    e. the x-ray beam is selectively filtered.

15. Computed tomography results in improved contrast resolution because
    a. digital techniques are employed.
    b. tissue superimposition is reduced.
    c. tissues are superimposed.
    d. precise beam collimation is employed.
    e. kVp is significantly increased.

16. The mathematics of back projection applied to image reconstruction in CT is credited to
    a. Alan Cormack.
    b. Raymond Damadian.
    c. Geodfrey Hounsfield.
    d. Frank Lauterbur.
    e. Perry Sprawls.

17. Place the following in chronological order.
    1. CT
    2. electron beam CT (EBCT)
    3. multisection computed tomography
    4. spiral CT

    a. 1, 2, 3, 4
    b. 1, 2, 4, 3
    c. 1, 3, 2, 4
    d. 1, 4, 2, 3
    e. 1, 3, 4, 2

18. The term "projection," when applied to CT, refers to
    a. speed of image acquisition.
    b. a data set representing x-ray attenuation in the patient.
    c. the size of the x-ray beam projected on the patient.
    d. the shape of the x-ray beam projected on the patient.
    e. the mathematics of image reconstruction.

19. Compared to projection radiography, conventional tomography will improve
    1. contrast resolution.
    2. patient dose.
    3. superimposition of tissues.
    4. spatial resolution.

    a. Only 1, 2, and 3 are correct.
    b. Only 1 and 3 are correct.
    c. Only 2 and 4 are correct.
    d. Only 4 is correct.
    e. All are correct.

20. Which of the following image modalities are likely to have less scatter radiation affecting the image?
    a. fluoroscopy
    b. projection of radiography
    c. conventional tomography
    d. CT
    e. radioisotope emission tomography

21. **What is the principal cause of reduced contrast in projection radiography?**
    a. useful beam radiation
    b. scatter radiation
    c. leakage radiation
    d. collimation
    e. kVp

22. **The first CT image was demonstrated by**
    a. Alan Cormack.
    b. Raymond Damadian.
    c. Geodfrey Hounsfield.
    d. Frank Lauterbur.
    e. Larry Rothenberg.

23. **The principal advantage of CT over conventional tomography is**
    a. speed of image acquisition.
    b. reduced patient dose.
    c. improved contrast resolution.
    d. improved spatial resolution.
    e. fewer artifacts.

24. **Which of the following imaging modalities appeared first?**
    a. emission imaging with radioisotopes
    b. diagnostic ultrasound
    c. projection radiography
    d. electron beam CT (EBCT)
    e. spiral CT

25. **Image presentation in conventional tomography is**
    a. axial.
    b. coronal.
    c. sagittal.
    d. transverse.
    e. volumetric.

26. **When compared to projection radiography, conventional tomography shows**
    a. better spatial resolution.
    b. less tissue superimposition.
    c. reduced patient dose.
    d. relaxed quality control.
    e. less operator involvement.

27. **Compared to CT, film/screen radiography will give**
    1. better spatial resolution.
    2. lower entrance surface dose for a single image.
    3. lower tube heating for a single image.
    4. better low contrast resolution.

    a. Only 1, 2, and 3 are correct.
    b. Only 1 and 3 are correct.
    c. Only 2 and 4 are correct.
    d. Only 4 is correct.
    e. All are correct.

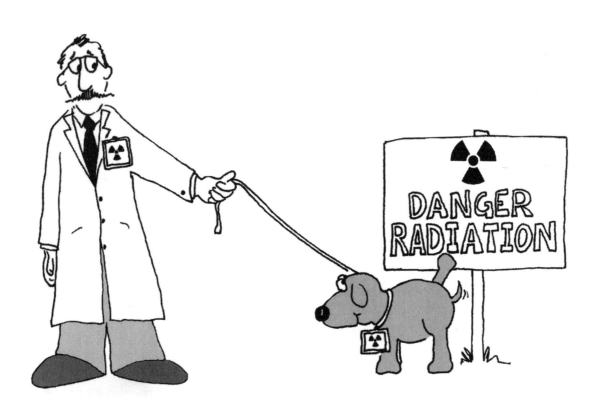

Operational Modes

- The major early computed tomography (CT) developments were given the misnomer **generation**, as in genealogy.

- Progress was rapid so that fourth-generation CT imagers appeared in 1978, just 6 years after the first CT imager.

- Unlike Hounsfield's early experiments, the patient does not move during CT, except for spiral CT, rather, the x-ray source and the image receptor move.

FIRST GENERATION

- Finely collimated x-ray beam (pencil beam) was used in first-generation CT imagers.

- Fan-shaped x-ray beam (fan beam) is used in all current CT imagers.

- Single radiation detector.

- Translate-rotate motion.

- 180 translations with 1° rotation between translations.

- Single image projection per translation.

- Five minute imaging time.

- Head imager only, not capable of body imaging.

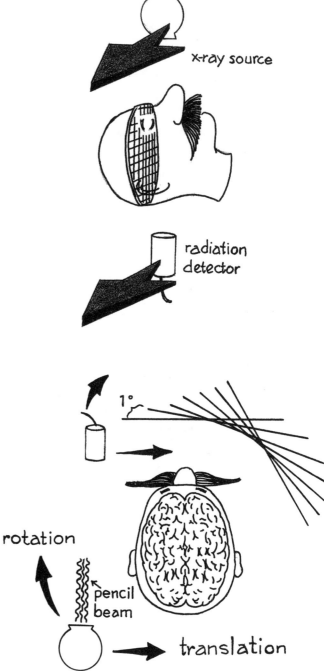

x-ray source

radiation detector

1°

rotation

pencil beam

translation

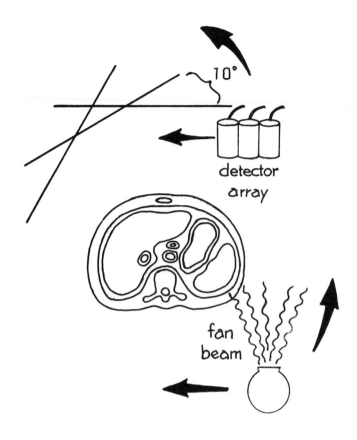

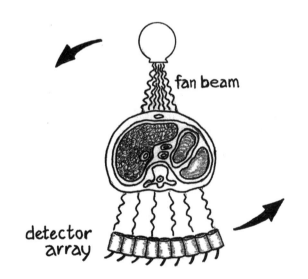

SECOND GENERATION

- Fan-shaped x-ray beam.

- Multiple radiation detectors—a **detector array**.

- Translate-rotate motion.

- Usually 18 translations with 10° rotation between translations.

- Multiple image projections per translation.

- Approximately, 30 s imaging time.

- Head and body imager.

THIRD GENERATION

- A fan beam x-ray source is used and it views the entire patient during imaging.

- As many as several hundred radiation detectors are incorporated into the **curvilinear** detector array.

- The curvilinear detector array provides constant distance between source and each detector, resulting in good image reconstruction.

- This development is based on 360° rotate-rotate motion. Both the x-ray source and the detector array rotate about the same axis.

- Hundreds of image projections are acquired during each rotation, resulting in better contrast resolution and spatial resolution.

- Imaging time is reduced to 1 s or less.

- Various arc scans are possible in order to improve motion blur—half scan, full scan.

- Ring artifacts are characteristic of third-generation imagers.

FOURTH GENERATION

- Fourth generation was developed principally to suppress ring artifacts.

- The x-ray source is collimated to a fan beam as in third generation.

- The detector array can contain several thousand individual detectors.

- The mechanical motion is rotation of the x-ray source around a fixed detector array (rotate-stationary).

- There is a modest sacrifice in geometry; however, the unattenuated leading edge and unattenuated trailing edge of the fan beam allows for individual detector calibration during each scan.

- Patient dose may be somewhat higher with fourth-generation scanners because of interspace between detectors.

- When there is an interspace between detectors, some x-radiation falls on the interspace, resulting in wasted dose.

- As the fan beam passes across each detector, an image projection is acquired.

- Imaging time is 1 s or less.

- Various arc scans are available—half scan, full scan, over scan.

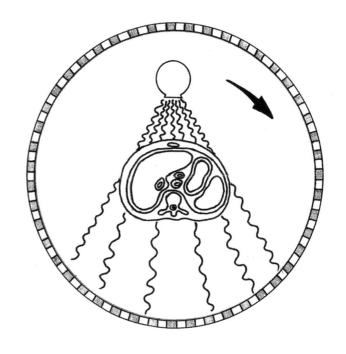

ELECTRON BEAM CT (EBCT)

- This CT imager was developed specifically for fast imaging.

- Images can be obtained in less than 100 ms, about the time of a radiograph.

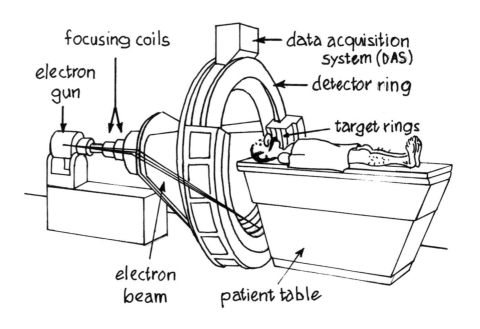

- The x-ray source is not an x-ray tube but rather a focussed, steered, and microwave-accelerated electron beam incident on a tungsten target.

- The target covers one-half of the imaging circle; the detector array covers the other half.

- The electron beam is steered along the curved tungsten target creating a moving source.

- There are four targets, or focal tracks, and four detector arrays, resulting in four contiguous images simultaneously.

- Electron beam CT is principally applied to cardiac imaging and frequently advertised as a **heart scan**.

- Electron beam CT has no moving parts.

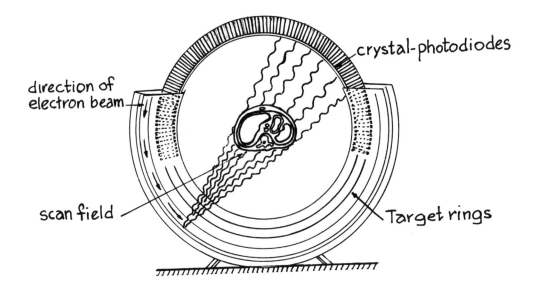

- Electron beam CT uses a focussed electron beam on a tungsten target ring as an x-ray source.

- Heat dissipation is no problem in EBCT.

- Electron beam CT can produce up to eight slices simultaneously.

- Electron beam CT scan times as short as 50 ms are possible.

- Principal application for EBCT is cardiac imaging.

SPIRAL CT

- Spiral CT was introduced to clinical practice in 1989 and is now the standard CT imager.

- If a third- or fourth-generation CT imager is caused to continually rotate while the patient couch is moved through the imaging plane, spiral CT results.

- The development of slip rings was the technology breakthrough that made spiral CT possible.

- Spiral CT requires slip ring technology for data transfer from the rotating gantry.

- Spiral CT requires either an on-board high-voltage supply so that coiled high-voltage cables are unnecessary or slip rings for high-voltage transfer.

- The principal advantage to spiral CT is the ability to image large volumes of anatomy in less time.

- Single breathhold imaging of the entire torso is possible with spiral CT.

	First generation 1972	Spiral CT 1999
scan time	300 s	< 1s
data/image	60 kB	2 MB
matrix size	80^2	1024^2
Energy/image	2 kJ	60 kJ
slice thickness	13 mm	1-10 mm
spatial resolution	3 lp/cm	15 lp/cm
contrast resolution @ 50 mGy	± 5 HU @ 5 mm	± 3 HU @ 3 mm

Chapter 2 Practice Questions

1. **Which of the following is characteristic of a first-generation CT imager?**

   a. detector array
   b. fan beam
   c. pencil beam
   d. rotate geometry
   e. slip ring technology

2. **Which of the following CT imagers is often referred to as the heart scan?**

   a. second generation
   b. third generation
   c. fourth generation
   d. electron beam
   e. spiral

3. **Which of the following is a particular characteristic of fourth-generation CT imagers?**

   a. fan x-ray beam geometry
   b. multielement detector array
   c. 1 s imaging time
   d. fixed detector array
   e. rotate-translate motion

4. Which of the following CT imagers has no mechanical moving parts in the gantry?

   a. second generation
   b. third generation
   c. fourth generation
   d. electron beam
   e. spiral

5. Which of the following is characteristic of a first-generation CT imager?

   a. detector array
   b. fan beam
   c. five minute imaging time
   d. rotate beam
   e. slip ring technology

6. Which of the following features led to the development of the spiral CT imager?

   a. megaheat unit x-ray tubes
   b. molybdenum/rhodium targeted x-ray tubes
   c. electronic slip rings
   d. high-frequency generators
   e. fast reconstruction algorithms

7. Ring artifacts are characteristic of

   a. first-generation CT.
   b. second-generation CT.
   c. third-generation CT.
   d. fourth-generation CT.
   e. spiral CT.

8. Which of the following is characteristic of a second-generation CT imager?

   a. able to image head only, not body
   b. five minute imaging time
   c. pencil-shaped x-ray beam
   d. single image projection per translation
   e. translate-rotate motion

9. The principal advantage to electron beam CT (EBCT) is

   a. imaging without x-rays.
   b. large volume imaging.
   c. one second imaging time.
   d. removal of ring artifacts.
   e. subsecond imaging time.

10. Which of the following is characteristic of a second-generation CT imager?

    a. able to image head only, not body
    b. five minute imaging time
    c. pencil-shaped x-ray beam
    d. single image projection per translation
    e. thirty second imaging time

11. During spiral CT, the motion of the patient couch is

    a. stationary.
    b. rotating.

   c. advanced step wise.

   d. alternating advance retreat.

   e. continuously advanced.

12. **Which of following are characteristic of a first-generation CT imager?**

   1. pencil beam

   2. single detector

   3. translate-rotate motion

   4. no body imaging

   a. Only 1, 2, and 3 are correct.

   b. Only 1 and 3 are correct.

   c. Only 2 and 4 are correct.

   d. Only 4 is correct.

   e. All are correct.

13. **Current design of electron beam CT (EBCT) allows for simultaneous production of**

   a. a single slice.

   b. two slices.

   c. four slices.

   d. eight slices.

   e. sixteen slices.

14. **Which of the following is characteristic of a second-generation CT imager?**

   1. fan-shaped x-ray beam

   2. detector array

   3. translate-rotate motion

   4. capable of imaging head and body

   a. Only 1, 2, and 3 are correct.

   b. Only 1 and 3 are correct.

   c. Only 2 and 4 are correct.

   d. Only 4 is correct.

   e. All are correct.

15. **X-radiation produced by an electron beam CT (EBCT) imager is emitted from a/an**

   a. electron plasma.

   b. electron tungsten plasma.

   c. rotating tungsten disk.

   d. rotating semicircular tungsten ring.

   e. fixed tungsten semicircular ring.

16. **Which of the following employ(s) fan beam geometry?**

   1. second-generation CT

   2. third-generation CT

   3. fourth-generation CT

   4. spiral CT

   a. Only 1, 2, and 3 are correct.

   b. Only 1 and 3 are correct.

   c. Only 2 and 4 are correct.

   d. Only 4 is correct.

   e. All are correct.

17. **Which of the following is characteristic of a third-generation CT imager?**

    a. pencil beam x-ray geometry
    b. single radiation detector
    c. curvilinear detector array
    d. 30 s imaging time
    e. single image projection per rotation

18. **The source of x-rays in an electron beam CT (EBCT) imager is a**

    a. high capacity fixed anode x-ray tube.
    b. high rotating anode x-ray tube.
    c. tungsten target ring.
    d. special molybdenum targeted x-ray tube.
    e. special molybdenum/rhodium targeted x-ray tube.

19. **One characteristic of a third-generation CT imager is**

    a. pencil x-ray beam.
    b. linear detector array.
    c. curvilinear detector array.
    d. 5 s imaging.
    e. single image projection per rotation.

20. **Which of the following is characteristic of a first-generation CT imager?**

    a. detector array
    b. fan beam
    c. rotate beam
    d. single image projection per translation
    e. slip ring technology

21. **A half-scan might be implemented during third-generation CT imaging in order to**

    a. improve spatial resolution.
    b. improve contrast resolution.
    c. reduce motion blur.
    d. reduce detector blur.
    e. allow higher technique.

22. **Which of the following CT imagers has a moving source of radiation?**

    1. second generation
    2. third generation
    3. fourth generation
    4. electron beam

    a. Only 1, 2, and 3 are correct.
    b. Only 1 and 2 are correct.
    c. Only 2 and 4 are correct.
    d. Only 4 is correct.
    e. All are correct.

23. **Which of the following are characteristic of a fourth-generation CT imager?**

    1. translate-rotate motion
    2. pencil beam
    3. linear detector array
    4. fixed detector array

   a. Only 1, 2, and 3 are correct.
   b. Only 1 and 3 are correct.
   c. Only 2 and 4 are correct.
   d. Only 4 is correct.
   e. All are correct.

24. Which of the following is characteristic of a first-generation CT imager?

   a. detector array
   b. fan beam
   c. rotate beam
   d. slip ring technology
   e. translate-rotate motion

25. Which of the following is characteristic of a second-generation CT imager?

   a. able to image head only, not body
   b. five minute imaging time
   c. multiple image projection per translation
   d. pencil-shaped x-ray beam
   e. single image projection per translation

26. The mechanical motion of the x-ray tube/detector array in a fourth-generation CT imager is

   a. translate-translate.
   b. translate-rotate.
   c. rotate-rotate.
   d. rotate-stationary.
   e. stationary-rotate.

27. Concerning CT,

   1. most CT units are now designed to obtain direct sagittal images.
   2. doubling the mA will reduce the "noise" by a factor of two.
   3. x-ray tubes are operated between 60 and 80 kVp.
   4. typical slice widths range from 1 to 10 mm.

   a. Only 1, 2, and 3 are correct.
   b. Only 1 and 3 are correct.
   c. Only 2 and 4 are correct.
   d. Only 4 is correct.
   e. All are correct.

28. Which of the following is characteristic of electron beam CT (EBCT)?

   a. can generate an effective spiral image detection
   b. requires an x-ray tube with excess of 5 MHU capacity
   c. is subject to annoying artifacts
   d. employs rotate-rotate geometry
   e. produces four contiguous images simultaneously

29. Of the following CT imagers, which is likely to have fastest scan time?

   a. second generation
   b. third generation
   c. fourth generation
   d. electron beam
   e. spiral

30. The principal advantage of third-generation over second-generation CT imagers is

    a. imaging without x-rays.
    b. large volume imaging.
    c. 1 s imaging time.
    d. removal of ring artifacts.
    e. subsecond imaging time.

31. Which of the following CT imagers does not use an x-ray tube?

    a. second generation
    b. third generation
    c. fourth generation
    d. spiral
    e. electron beam

32. Which of the following is the single feature that characterizes third-generation CT imaging?

    a. fast imaging time
    b. acquisition of simultaneous image projections
    c. rotate-rotate motion
    d. fan beam x-ray geometry
    e. curvilinear detector array

33. Which of the following is characteristic of a second-generation CT imager?

    1. translate-rotate motion
    2. five minute imaging time
    3. a detector array
    4. pencil x-ray beam

    a. Only 1, 2, and 3 are correct.
    b. Only 1 and 3 are correct.
    c. Only 2 and 4 are correct.
    d. Only 4 is correct.
    e. All are correct.

34. The principal advantage to spiral CT is

    a. subsecond imaging time.
    b. 1 s imaging time.
    c. removal of ring artifacts.
    d. large volume imaging.
    e. imaging without x-rays.

35. When compared to third-generation, fourth-generation CT imagers usually have

    a. higher patient dose.
    b. better spatial resolution.
    c. better contrast resolution.
    d. more noise.
    e. more artifacts.

36. Which of the following is characteristic of a first-generation CT imager?
    a. detector array
    b. fan beam
    c. rotate beam
    d. single radiation detector
    e. slip ring technology

37. Which image artifact is characteristic of third-generation CT imagers?
    a. beam hardening
    b. motion
    c. ring
    d. spoke
    e. streak

38. In an electron beam CT (EBCT) imager the radiation used to produce the image is a
    a. fixed electron.
    b. fixed x-ray beam.
    c. mixed beam of electrons and x-rays.
    d. scanned electron beam.
    e. scanned x-ray beam.

39. Which of the following CT imagers is not limited by x-ray target heat dissipation?
    a. second generation
    b. third generation
    c. fourth generation
    d. electron beam
    e. spiral

40. Which of the following is characteristic of a first-generation CT imager?
    1. fan-shaped x-ray beam
    2. detector array
    3. 30 s imaging time
    4. single image projection per translation

    a. Only 1, 2, and 3 are correct.
    b. Only 1 and 3 are correct.
    c. Only 2 and 4 are correct.
    d. Only 4 is correct.
    e. All are correct.

41. Which of the following CT imagers is capable of 50 ms imaging time?
    a. second generation
    b. third generation
    c. fourth generation
    d. electron beam
    e. spiral

42. **Which of the following CT imagers finds principal application in cardiac imaging?**
    a. second generation
    b. third generation
    c. fourth generation
    d. spiral
    e. electron beam

43. **Which of the following is characteristic of a second-generation CT imager?**
    a. able to image head only, not body
    b. fan-shaped x-ray beam
    c. five minute imaging time
    d. pencil-shaped x-ray beam
    e. single image projection per translation

44. **Place the following CT imagers chronologically in the order of their introduction.**
    1. third generation
    2. spiral
    3. multisection
    4. electron beam

    a. 1, 2, 3, 4
    b. 1, 3, 4, 2
    c. 1, 4, 2, 3
    d. 4, 1, 2, 3
    e. 4, 3, 1, 2

45. **Which of the following is characteristic of a second-generation CT imager?**
    a. pencil-shaped x-ray beam
    b. capable of imaging head and body
    c. five minute imaging time
    d. able to image head only, not body
    e. single image projection per translation

46. **Which of the following CT imagers requires that the gantry have an on-board rotating high-voltage generator?**
    a. third generation
    b. fourth generation
    c. electron beam
    d. spiral
    e. multislice

47. **Which of the following CT imagers is capable of a scan time of 100 ms?**
    a. second generation
    b. third generation
    c. fourth generation
    d. electron beam
    e. spiral

48. **The principal advantage of fourth-generation over second-generation CT imagers is**

    a. imaging without x-rays.
    b. large volume imaging.
    c. 1 s imaging time.
    d. removal of ring artifacts.
    e. subsecond imaging time.

49. **The image receptor for a fourth-generation CT imager is**

    a. a multielement solid state detector array.
    b. a multielement linear detector array.
    c. a fixed detector array.
    d. 50-100 detectors.
    e. sodium iodine crystal detectors.

50. **Which of the following is characteristic of a second-generation CT imager?**

    a. a detector array
    b. able to image head only, not body
    c. five minute imaging time
    d. pencil-shaped x-ray beam
    e. single image projection per translation

51. **Which of the following CT imagers allows imaging of the entire thorax in one breathhold?**

    a. third generation
    b. fourth generation
    c. electron beam
    d. spiral
    e. multislice

52. **Concerning CT,**

    1. first-generation CT imagers had scan times of about 20 s.
    2. all CT imagers sold today are fourth-generation units.
    3. typical scan times of current CT imagers are in the range of 2 to 10 s.
    4. typical slice widths range from 1 to 10 mm.

    a. Only 1, 2, and 3 are correct.
    b. Only 1 and 3 are correct.
    c. Only 2 and 4 are correct.
    d. Only 4 is correct.
    e. All are correct.

53. **When compared to third-generation, fourth-generation CT imagers**

    a. have rotate-rotate mechanical motion.
    b. allow for individual detector calibration each scan.
    c. calibrate a reference detector each scan.
    d. have better contrast resolution.
    e. have better temporal resolution.

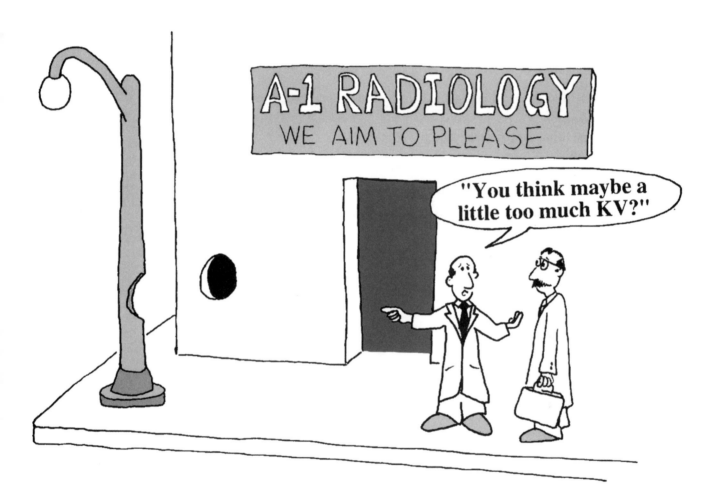

The CT Gantry

- Every computed tomography (CT) imager has three distinguishing components—the operating console, the computer, and the gantry.

- The operating console performs two major functions—imaging control with preselected technique conditions and image viewing and manipulation.

- There may be several operating consoles, each dedicated to a separate function, such as CT control or postprocessing and image analysis.

- The CT computer has no physically distinguishing features.

- The CT computer has high capacity and is very fast due to the large number of computations required on an extensive data set.

- Some CT imagers have the computer built into the operating console.

- Computers capable of multiprocessing are used in CT.

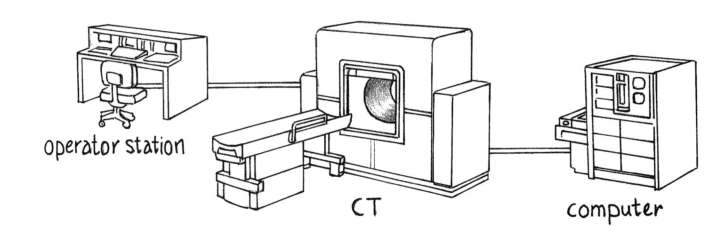

operator station CT computer

- Multiprocessing allows a computer to perform several functions at the same time, which reduces reconstruction time and increases capacity.

- The gantry is special to CT. It houses the x-ray source, the detector array, the collimator assembly, and, maybe, also the high-voltage generator.

- The patient aperture of a CT gantry has maximum diameter of approximately 70 cm.

- The CT gantry can be tilted either way approximately ±30°.

THE X-RAY SOURCE

- Computed tomography imaging places two demands on an x-ray tube—high x-ray intensity and rapid heat dissipation.

- High x-ray intensity is accomplished with a high mA generator and a generous focal spot size, up to 2 mm.

- Rapid heat dissipation is provided by large diameter, thick anode disks rotating at 10,000 rpm.

- X-ray tubes developed for CT have very high heat capacity.

- Anode heat capacity of 6 MHU (million heat units) are common. That compares to less than 1 MHU for general radiography.

- The anode-cathode axis is perpendicular to the patient axis to avoid the **heel effect**.

- Computed tomography x-ray tubes have high-speed (10,000 rpm) rotors.

- X-ray tube failure is the principal cause of CT imager malfunction.

- X-ray tube current of 200 to 800 mA are common. Too low mA can result in unacceptable image noise.

- X-ray tube potential is usually 120 kVp to 140 kVp three phase or high frequency.

- Such high kVp is used for higher intensity and penetrability, and therefore, less x-ray tube loading and lower patient dose.

single phase

$$1\,HU = 1\,kV_p \times 1\,mA \times 1s$$

three phase / high frequency

$$1\,HU = 1.4 \times 1\,kV_p \times 1\,mA \times 1s$$

$$1\,HU = 1\,kV \times 1\,mA \times 1s$$
$$1\,HU = 1\,V \times 1\,A \times 1s$$
$$1\,V = 1\,J/C$$
$$1\,A = 1\,C/s$$
$$1\,HU = 1\,J/C \times 1\,C/s \times 1s$$
$$1\,HU = 1\,J$$

- Dual focus tubes are common, usually having 0.5 and 1.0 mm focal spots, with the smaller focal spot used for better spatial resolution.

- The improved spatial resolution does not result from projection geometry as in radiography, rather from better x-ray beam—radiation detector collimation.

- Still, the principal effect on spatial resolution is matrix size and field of view (FOV).

- For third-generation CT imagers, the x-ray source is pulsed. Each pulse creates an image projection from each detector.

- When pulsed, up to 100 mA is used with pulse widths of 1 to 5 ms at pulse repetition rates of 60 Hz.

- For fourth-generation imagers the x-ray tube is energized continuously.

- Each pass of a fourth-generation fan beam over a detector produces an image projection.

- Computed tomography x-ray beams are filtered to harden the beam and make it more uniform at the detector array.

- Filtration produces a higher energy, more homogeneous x-ray beam and reduces the beam-hardening artifact (see Chapter 8).

- A shaped x-ray beam filter is used in CT to produce a more uniform intensity at the detector array.

- A "bow tie" filter is often used to even radiation intensity at the detector array.

HIGH-VOLTAGE GENERATOR

- High kVp is used to minimize photoelectric absorption and, therefore, patient dose.

- High kVp is used to reduce bone attenuation relative to soft tissue allowing a wider dynamic range of the image.

- High kVp is used to increase radiation intensity at the detector array.

- High kVp is used to reduce x-ray tube loading, because of lower mA and thereby, extend tube life.

- Three phase or high-frequency voltage generation is used for CT imagers.

Typical technique :
125 kVp/400mA/2s = 100 k HU

Q: How much heat energy is produced by 15 100ms images acquired at 130 kVp/600mA?

A: 15 × 0.1s × 130 kVp × 600mA = 0.2 MJ

- Three phase voltage is usually generated by a stand alone module near the gantry. Cables that will only wind 360° must be used, causing reversal of gantry rotation.

- High-frequency generators are small enough that they can be mounted on the rotating gantry.

- Heat units (HU) and joules (J) are equivalent measures of energy.

- Slip rings make possible continuous rotation of the x-ray source leading to spiral CT.

- Slip rings incorporate circular electrical conductors, one type of which rotates and passes power to the high-voltage generator; the other passes signals from the data acquisition system (DAS) to the computer.

- Three phase power was used until mid 1980s.

- Essentially all CT imagers now use high-frequency generators.

- The high-frequency generator can be positioned on the rotating gantry with the x-ray source.

- The high-frequency generator can be positioned on the fixed part of the gantry and connected to the x-ray source through slip rings.

- The DAS is located between the detector array and the computer.

- The DAS (1) amplifies the detector signal; (2) converts the analog signal to digital (ADC); and (3) transmits the digital signal to the computer.

- High-frequency voltage generation eliminates the need for massive high-voltage transformers.

slip ring technology allows:
- faster imaging
- no interscan delay
- continuous data acquisition
- continuous imaging .. no start-stop
- no cable wrap

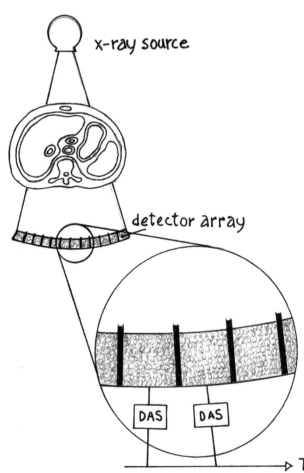

x-ray source

detector array

DAS   DAS

→ To computer

DETECTOR ARRAY

- The evolution of the CT radiation detector has progressed with continuous improvements.

- Detector efficiency is important because it determines maximum tube loading and controls patient dose.

- Three important features of the detector array are efficiency, number of detectors, and detector concentration.

- Early CT imagers used a scintillation crystal-photomultiplier tube as a single element detector.

- A grouping of detectors is called a **detector array**.

- There are two types of detector arrays—gas-filled and solid state.

- Gas-filled detectors—high-pressure xenon—have very fast response and no afterglow but only about 50% detection efficiency.

- Gas-filled detectors can be packed more tightly than solid state detectors with less interspace septa.

- Most solid state detectors today use a scintillator, cadmium tungstate ($CdWO_4$), optically coupled to a photodiode.

- Solid state detectors have nearly 100% detection efficiency but cannot be tightly packed.

- The detector array consists of many individual detectors fashioned as a module that are positioned on a receptor board for easy exchange and service.

- A gas-filled detector array uses small ion chambers filled with high-pressure xenon or other gas.

- Each ion chamber is about 1 mm wide with essentially no interspace.

- The geometric efficiency—the percent area of the detector array that is detector, not interspace—is more than 90%.

detector	signal source
NaI	PMT
Xe	ion chambers
CsI	photodiode
BGO	photodiode
$CdWO_4$	photodiode

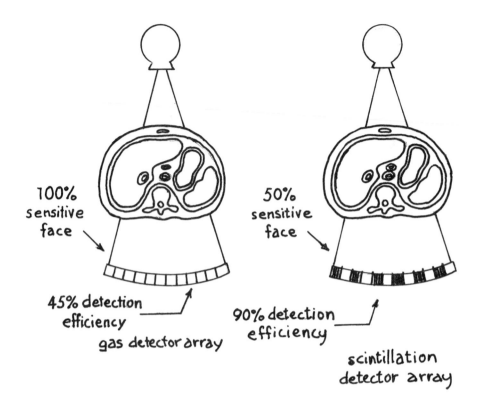

100%
sensitive
face

50%
sensitive
face

45% detection
efficiency

gas detector array

90% detection
efficiency

scintillation
detector array

- The intrinsic detection efficiency for high-pressure xenon is approximately 50%.

- Total detector efficiency = geometric efficiency × intrinsic efficiency.

- Solid state detectors are made of a scintillation crystal, which when irradiated emits light that is converted to an analog signal by a photodiode.

- Solid state detectors have approximately 90% intrinsic detection efficiency. Essentially, all incident x-rays are detected.

- Total detection efficiency depends on the number of detectors and how tightly they are packed.

- When there is interspace between detectors, detection efficiency is reduced and patient dose increased.

- Eighty percent total detection efficiency is common for solid state detector arrays.

- Solid state detectors are automatically recalibrated between scans.

- Solid state detectors are more expensive than gas-filled detectors and their increased efficiency can result in less x-ray tube loading, reduced image noise and reduced patient dose.

- The DAS is positioned just after the detector array to amplify each signal, and properly sequence each signal to the computer.

- Multiple detector arrays allow the collection of two or more image data sets simultaneously.

- Multiple detector arrays can reduce heat loading of the x-ray tube.

- Multiple detector arrays allow simultaneous imaging of two or more slices.

COLLIMATOR ASSEMBLY

- There are two collimators in CT—**prepatient** and **postpatient**.

- The prepatient collimator is positioned near the x-ray source.

- The prepatient collimator controls patient dose and determines the dose profile.

- As the prepatient collimator is narrowed, patient dose increases and the dose profile becomes more rounded.

- Prepatient collimation controls patient dose profile.

- Postpatient collimation controls slice thickness.

- The dose profile is a plot of dose across the slice thickness.

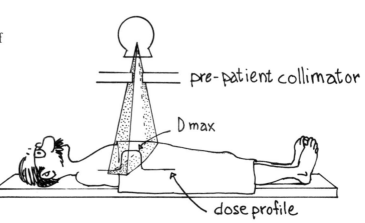

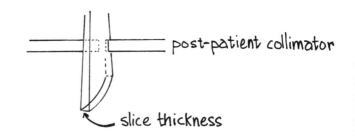

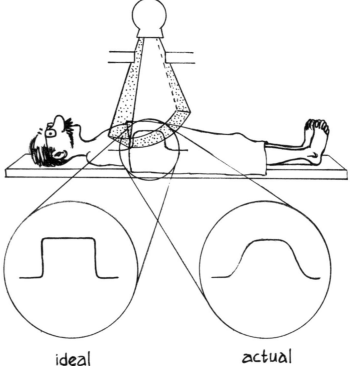

ideal   actual

$$\text{Voxel size } (mm^3) = \frac{FOV}{matrix} \times \text{slice thickness}$$

Q: What is the voxel size for a 2 mm slice thickness imaged with a 320 x 320 matrix over a 20 cm field of view?

A: $\frac{200\,mm^2}{320} \times 2\,mm = 1.25\,mm^3$

- The dose profile should be square but is rounded because of scatter radiation.

- The postpatient collimator controls slice thickness (sensitivity profile).

- When the postpatient collimators are narrowed, slice thickness is reduced.

- Sensitivity profile is a plot of detector response versus distance (mm).

- The ideal sensitivity profile is square; in practice, it is rounded because of scatter radiation.

- Prepatient and postpatient collimators are controlled together to match dose profile and sensitivity profile.

- If dose profile exceeds sensitivity profile, patient dose is excessive.

- If sensitivity profile exceeds dose profile, image quality is compromised.

- Nominal slice thickness is controllable between approximately 1 and 10 mm.

- As the slice thickness is changed, so is the voxel size.

- Thinner slices are required for rapidly changing anatomy, for example, the inner ear.

- Thinner slices result in less partial volume effect.

- Thinner slices result in improved spatial resolution.

- Thinner slices result in higher patient dose because of increased overlap of slices.

- When imaging with thin slices they are usually contiguous so that no tissue is missed.

- High-voltage slip rings are oil-insulated and transfer power from an external high-voltage generator to the gantry.

- Low-voltage slip rings are air-insulated and transfer data from gantry to computer.

- When a spiral CT is based on low-voltage slip rings, the high-voltage generator is high-frequency type and mounted on the rotating gantry.

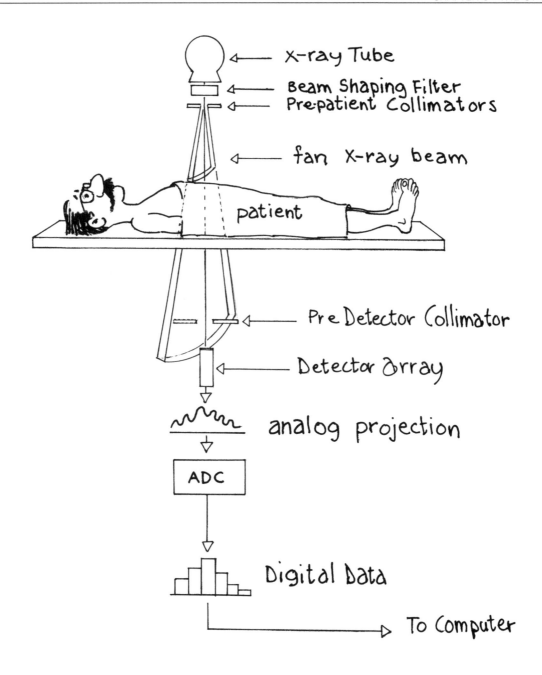

Chapter 3 Practice Questions

1. **Which of the following represents the three principal components of a CT imager?**

    a. patient couch, gantry, high-voltage generator
    b. gantry, operating console, computer
    c. operating console, patient couch, high-voltage generator
    d. computer, high-voltage generator, operating console
    e. reconstruction apparatus, operating console, patient couch

2. The principal function(s) of the operating console is (are)
   1. control of image acquisition.
   2. image reconstruction.
   3. image viewing and manipulation.
   4. patient positioning.

   a. Only 1, 2, and 3 are correct.
   b. Only 1 and 3 are correct.
   c. Only 2 and 4 are correct.
   d. Only 4 is correct.
   e. All are correct.

3. Postprocessing of an image is possible principally because of the
   a. operating console.
   b. CT computer.
   c. CT gantry.
   d. display console.
   e. operating keyboard.

4. A 24-cm field of view (FOV) is imaged using a 512 matrix, what is the pixel size?
   a. 0.25 mm
   b. 0.5 mm
   c. 0.75 mm
   d. 1.09 mm
   e. 1.25 mm

5. The maximum diameter of the patient aperture in a CT imager is approximately
   a. 40 cm.
   b. 50 cm.
   c. 70 cm.
   d. 90 cm.
   e. 120 cm.

6. In order to perform transverse oblique CT imaging, the
   a. patient couch can be tilted plus or minus 10 degrees.
   b. patient couch can be tilted plus or minus 30 degrees.
   c. gantry can be tilted plus or minus 10 degrees.
   d. gantry can be tilted plus or minus 30 degrees.
   e. gantry can be rotated.

7. Two principal demands placed on an x-ray tube for CT imaging are
   a. heat dissipation and beam filtration.
   b. high x-ray intensity and heat dissipation.
   c. high x-ray intensity and rotation speed.
   d. line focus principle and rotating anode.
   e. reduced focal spot size and heat dissipation.

8. Which of the following characteristics contributes to high x-ray intensity in a CT x-ray tube?

   1. large focal spot size
   2. high speed rotor
   3. high mA generator
   4. massive anode

   a. Only 1, 2, and 3 are correct.
   b. Only 1 and 3 are correct.
   c. Only 2 and 4 are correct.
   d. Only 4 is correct.
   e. All are correct.

9. One hundred heat units (HU) is equivalent to

   a. 1 erg.
   b. 100 erg.
   c. 1 joule (J).
   d. 100 joule (J).
   e. 100 coulomb per kilogram.

10. Which of the following characteristics contributes to heat dissipation in a CT x-ray tube?

    a. high-frequency generator
    b. increased beam filtration
    c. large diameter disk
    d. precise beam collimation
    e. small focal spot

11. Which of the following is a function of the data acquisition system (DAS)?

    1. amplify the detected signal
    2. convert the detected signal to analog form
    3. transmit the detected signal to the computer
    4. postprocess the detected signal

    a. Only 1, 2, and 3 are correct.
    b. Only 1 and 3 are correct.
    c. Only 2 and 4 are correct.
    d. Only 4 is correct.
    e. All are correct.

12. Which of the following is a principal characteristic of x-ray tubes developed specifically for CT?

    a. small focal spot
    b. small size
    c. high heat capacity
    d. high generator capacity
    e. ability to rotate

13. One advantage to using high kVp during CT imaging is the reduction in

    a. image time.
    b. image reconstruction time.
    c. radiation intensity at the image receptor.
    d. patient dose.
    e. x-ray tube loading.

14. **Which of the following describes the x-ray tube used for CT?**

    a. It is positioned with the anode-cathode axis perpendicular to the patient axis
    b. It is positioned with the anode-cathode axis parallel with the patient axis
    c. It has heat capacity of at least 1 MHU
    d. The rotor speed is fixed at 3600 rpm
    e. Most heat is dissipated by convection

15. **Which of the following currently are employed as the detectors in the CT imager?**

    1. crystal-photomultiplier
    2. ion chamber
    3. Geiger counter
    4. crystal-photodiode

    a. Only 1, 2, and 3 are correct.
    b. Only 1 and 3 are correct.
    c. Only 2 and 4 are correct.
    d. Only 4 is correct.
    e. All are correct.

16. **Which of the following is the principal cause of failure of a CT imager?**

    a. high-voltage generator failure
    b. operating console failure
    c. patient couch failure
    d. radiation detector failure
    e. x-ray tube failure

17. **Which of the following is characteristic of a CT imager?**

    1. imaging time of 0.1-1 s
    2. image reconstruction time of 5-10 s
    3. x-ray tube current of 200-800 mA
    4. x-ray tube potential of 60-100 kVp

    a. Only 1, 2, and 3 are correct.
    b. Only 1 and 3 are correct.
    c. Only 2 and 4 are correct.
    d. Only 4 is correct.
    e. All are correct.

18. **A useful characteristic of a gas-filled detector for CT imaging is**

    a. no afterglow.
    b. high detection efficiency.
    c. response integration.
    d. direct digitation.
    e. data acquisition system (DAS) not required.

19. **The principal reason that high kVp is employed in CT imaging is reduced**

    a. scan time.
    b. reconstruction time.
    c. patient dose.
    d. image noise.
    e. image latitude.

20. The number of heat units (HU) in CT imaging is
    a. 1 kVp × 1 mA.
    b. 1 kVp × 1 mA x1 s.
    c. 1.4 × 1 kVp × 1 mA.
    d. 1.4 × 1 kVp × 1 mA × 1 s.
    e. 2.8 × 1 kVp × 1 mA × 1 s.

21. If dose profile exceeds section sensitivity profile, what suffers most?
    a. contrast resolution
    b. image artifacts
    c. image noise
    d. patient dose
    e. spatial resolution

22. Which of the following is characteristic of a CT imager?
    a. fixed anode x-ray tube
    b. single focus x-ray tube (0.5 mm)
    c. single focus x-ray tube (1 mm)
    d. dual focus x-ray tube (0.1 and 0.5 mm)
    e. dual focus x-ray tube (0.5 and 1 mm)

23. When using a dual focus x-ray tube for CT imaging, the smaller focal spot is employed to improve
    a. patient dose.
    b. image contrast.
    c. spatial resolution.
    d. image noise.
    e. imaging time.

24. Which of the following principally controls pixel size?
    1. prepatient collimation
    2. field of view (FOV)
    3. postpatient collimation
    4. matrix size

    a. Only 1, 2, and 3 are correct.
    b. Only 1 and 3 are correct.
    c. Only 2 and 4 are correct.
    d. Only 4 is correct.
    e. All is correct.

25. Third-generation CT imagers employ
    a. <100 kVp.
    b. either pulsed beam or pulsed detector interrogation.
    c. fixed anode x-ray tubes.
    d. lower mA than second generation.
    e. pulsed radiation detectors.

26. An image projection is the
    a. image encoded in the remnant x-ray beam.
    b. latent image in computer space.
    c. reconstructed image.
    d. signal acquired by each detector.
    e. use of binary code to digitize the image.

27. The scintillator used in most CT imager detectors is

    a. sodium iodide.
    b. xenon.
    c. cesium iodide.
    d. calcium tungstate.
    e. cadmium tungstate.

28. A typical CT imaging technique involves 120 kVp, 600 mA, 1 s. The total heat units (HU) generated are approximately

    a. 50 kHU.
    b. 100 kHU.
    c. 200 kHU.
    d. 300 kHU.
    e. 500 kHU.

29. A high-pressure xenon detector array has the following characteristics: (1) 95% geometric efficiency; (2) 45% intrinsic efficiency. What is the total detection efficiency?

    a. 43%
    b. 45%
    c. 57%
    d. 92%
    e. 95%

30. A typical imaging technique for spiral CT is 130 kVp, 200 mA for 15 s. The total heat generated is approximately

    a. 400 kHU.
    b. 450 kHU.
    c. 500 kHU.
    d. 550 kHU.
    e. 600 kHU.

31. In a detector array, the larger the interspace between detectors the greater will be

    a. afterglow.
    b. data acquisition system (DAS) time.
    c. image reconstruction.
    d. patient dose.
    e. response time.

32. Which of the following principally influences the dose profile?

    a. data acquisition system (DAS)
    b. detector response time
    c. postpatient collimator
    d. prepatient collimator
    e. section sensitivity

33. The principal reason to filter the x-ray beam of a CT imager is to

    a. reduce patient dose.
    b. homogenize the beam at the detector array.
    c. equalize beam intensity at the detector array.
    d. reduce imaging time.
    e. remove image artifacts.

34. **The shaped x-ray beam filter used in many CT scanners is termed a/an**
    a. belt.
    b. bow tie.
    c. detector.
    d. slip.
    e. uniform.

35. **Which component of the CT imager principally controls section sensitivity profile?**
    a. prepatient collimator
    b. postpatient collimator
    c. beam filtration
    d. shaped beam filter
    e. data acquisition system (DAS)

36. **Which of the following is often termed the "predetector collimator"?**
    a. prepatient collimation
    b. postpatient collimation
    c. prepatient filter
    d. postpatient filter
    e. detector interspace

37. **Which improvements followed the introduction of slip ring technology?**
    1. continuous imaging
    2. no interscan delay
    3. continuous data acquisition
    4. faster imaging

    a. Only 1, 2, and 3 are correct.
    b. Only 1 and 3 are correct.
    c. Only 2 and 4 are correct.
    d. Only 4 is correct.
    e. All are correct.

38. **Which of the following is helpful in reducing partial volume artifacts?**
    1. reduce field of view (FOV)
    2. reduce matrix size
    3. prepatient collimation
    4. postpatient collimation

    a. Only 1, 2, and 3 are correct.
    b. Only 1 and 3 are correct.
    c. Only 2 and 4 are correct.
    d. Only 4 is correct.
    e. All are correct.

39. **By employing high kVp for CT imaging, one can reduce**
    a. Compton scatter.
    b. patient dose.
    c. image artifacts.
    d. image reconstruction time.
    e. imaging time.

40. **The purpose of using high kVp for CT imaging is reduced**

    a. photoelectric absorption.
    b. Compton scatter.
    c. imaging time.
    d. image reconstruction time.
    e. patient dose.

41. **Aluminum filtration will have the greatest effect on which CT image property?**

    a. CT number
    b. spatial resolution
    c. contrast
    d. noise
    e. temporal resolution

42. **Which of the following is a function of the data acquisition system (DAS)?**

    1. convert the power to high frequency
    2. convert the detected signal to digital form
    3. postprocess the detected signal
    4. transmit the detected signal to the computer

    a. Only 1, 2, and 3 are correct.
    b. Only 1 and 3 are correct.
    c. Only 2 and 4 are correct.
    d. Only 4 is correct.
    e. All are correct.

43. **When postpatient collimation is reduced, the result is**

    1. thinner section sensitivity profile.
    2. increased patient dose.
    3. less partial volume artifact.
    4. increased image noise.

    a. Only 1, 2, and 3 are correct.
    b. Only 1 and 3 are correct.
    c. Only 2 and 4 are correct.
    d. Only 4 is correct.
    e. All are correct.

44. **Which of the following is increased by the use of high kVp during CT imaging?**

    1. photoelectric absorption
    2. x-ray tube loading
    3. image dynamic range
    4. radiation intensity at the image receptor

    a. Only 1, 2, and 3 are correct.
    b. Only 1 and 3 are correct.
    c. Only 2 and 4 are correct.
    d. Only 4 is correct.
    e. All are correct.

45. A 320 by 320 matrix displays how many pixels?

    a. 320
    b. 640
    c. 960
    d. 102,400
    e. 32,768,000

46. Which of the following is the high-voltage employed in CT imaging?

    1. single phase half-wave rectified
    2. single phase full-wave rectified
    3. three phase half-wave rectified
    4. high frequency

    a. Only 1, 2, and 3 are correct.
    b. Only 1 and 3 are correct.
    c. Only 2 and 4 are correct.
    d. Only 4 is correct.
    e. Only are correct.

47. A 16-cm field of view (FOV) is imaged using a 320 matrix, what is the pixel size?

    a. 0.25 mm
    b. 0.5 mm
    c. 0.75 mm
    d. 1.0 mm
    e. 1.25 mm

48. Which of the following has/have been used in a solid state detector array for CT imaging?

    1. sodium iodide
    2. cesium iodide
    3. cadmium tungstate
    4. calcium tungstate

    a. Only 1, 2, and 3 are correct.
    b. Only 1 and 3 are correct.
    c. Only 2 and 4 are correct.
    d. Only 4 is correct.
    e. All are correct.

49. Which of the following characteristics contributes to heat dissipation in a CT x-ray tube?

    a. high-frequency generator
    b. increased beam filtration
    c. precise beam collimation
    d. small focal spot
    e. thick anode

50. Slip rings are employed in spiral CT to conduct
    1. high voltage.
    2. the x-ray beam.
    3. detector signals.
    4. the patient couch.

    a. Only 1, 2, and 3 are correct.
    b. Only 1 and 3 are correct.
    c. Only 2 and 4 are correct.
    d. Only 4 is correct.
    e. All are correct.

51. For a CT imager manufactured after 1995, which is the most likely source of high voltage?
    a. single phase half-wave rectified
    b. single phase full-wave rectified
    c. three phase 6 pulse
    d. three phase 12 pulse
    e. high frequency

52. A CT imager produces 20 images at a technique of 120 kVp, 400 mA, 1.5 s. What is the approximate heat load on the anode?
    a. 1.4 MJ
    b. 1.6 MJ
    c. 1.8 MJ
    d. 2.0 MJ
    e. 2.5 MJ

53. Conceptually, which component of the CT imager is located between the detector array and the computer?
    a. postprocessing computer
    b. the data acquisition system (DAS)
    c. the high-frequency generator
    d. the postpatient collimators
    e. the x-ray tube

54. Which of the following characteristics contributes to heat dissipation in a CT x-ray tube?
    a. high-speed rotor
    b. small focal spot
    c. high-frequency generator
    d. increased beam filtration
    e. precise beam collimation

55. Anode heat capacity of an x-ray tube designed for CT should have at least
    a. 100 kHU.
    b. 1 MHU.
    c. 5 MHU.
    d. 10 MHU.
    e. 20 MHU.

56. Each of the following helps control patient dose except:
    a. detector efficiency
    b. high-voltage generation
    c. imaging time
    d. patient couch incrementation
    e. postpatient collimation

57. Which of the following components **must** be on the rotating part of the CT gantry?
    a. array processor
    b. central processing unit
    c. detector array
    d. reconstruction kernal
    e. x-ray tube

58. A useful characteristic of a gas-filled detector for CT imaging is
    a. direct digital signal.
    b. extended afterglow.
    c. good energy dependence.
    d. high efficiency of detection.
    e. fast response time.

59. Which of the following is characteristic of a CT imager?
    a. scan times of 0.1-1 s
    b. image reconstruction times of 5-10 s
    c. x-ray tube current of 50-100 mA
    d. x-ray tube potential of 60-100 kVp
    e. focal spot size of 0.5 mm

60. Which of following is positioned near the x-ray source?
    1. beam filters
    2. data acquisition system (DAS)
    3. prepatient collimation
    4. postpatient collimation

    a. Only 1, 2, and 3 are correct.
    b. Only 1 and 3 are correct.
    c. Only 2 and 4 are correct.
    d. Only 4 is correct.
    e. All are correct.

61. The principal reason that high kVp is employed in CT imaging is
    a. reduced scan time.
    b. reduced reconstruction time.
    c. increased beam penetrability.
    d. reduced image noise.
    e. reduced image latitude.

62. Which of the following is/are positive characteristics of solid state detector arrays?

    1. very fast response time
    2. no afterglow
    3. high geometric detection efficiency
    4. high intrinsic detection efficiency

    a. Only 1, 2, and 3 are correct.
    b. Only 1 and 3 are correct.
    c. Only 2 and 4 are correct.
    d. Only 4 is correct.
    e. All are correct.

63. One heat unit (HU) is equal to

    a. 100 erg.
    b. 1 joule (J).
    c. 100 rad.
    d. 1 joule (J) per coulomb.
    e. 1 coulomb per second.

64. A solid state detector array has the following characteristics: (1) 40% geometric detection efficiency; (2) 90% intrinsic detection efficiency. What is the total detector efficiency?

    a. 36%
    b. 40%
    c. 57%
    d. 87%
    e. 90%

65. A 40-cm field of view (FOV) is imaged using a 512 matrix and 5 mm slice thickness, what is the approximate voxel size?

    a. 1 mm^3
    b. 2 mm^3
    c. 3 mm^3
    d. 4 mm^3
    e. 5 mm^3

66. When comparing high-pressure gas-filled detectors with solid state detectors, gas-filled detectors

    1. have higher geometric efficiency.
    2. have higher intrinsic efficiency.
    3. respond faster.
    4. have higher afterglow.

    a. Only 1, 2, and 3 are correct.
    b. Only 1 and 3 are correct.
    c. Only 2 and 4 are correct.
    d. Only 4 is correct.
    e. All are correct.

67. A 16-cm field of view (FOV) is imaged using a 320 matrix and 10 mm slice thickness, what is the voxel size?

   a. 1 mm^3
   b. 2 mm^3
   c. 3 mm^3
   d. 4 mm^3
   e. 5 mm^3

68. The total detection efficiency of CT detector arrays is equal to

   a. geometric detection efficiency divided by intrinsic detection efficiency.
   b. intrinsic detection efficiency divided by geometric detection efficiency.
   c. intrinsic detection efficiency multiplied by geometric detection efficiency.
   d. intrinsic detection efficiency multiplied by response time.
   e. response time multiplied by geometric efficiency.

69. A multislice CT image is obtained at 130 kVp, 800 mA, 4 s. The resulting anode heat load is approximately

   a. 600 kHU.
   b. 700 kHU.
   c. 800 kHU.
   d. 900 kHU.
   e. 1 MHU.

70. As the interspace distance between detectors is reduced,

   a. detector response time is reduced.
   b. geometric efficiency is reduced.
   c. patient dose is increased.
   d. signal acquisition time is increased.
   e. total detector efficiency is increased.

71. The principal application of multidetector arrays is

   a. reduced patient dose.
   b. multiple simultaneous images.
   c. reduced image noise.
   d. improved spatial resolution.
   e. improved contrast resolution.

72. Which of the following are found in most CT imagers?

   1. beam filters
   2. prepatient collimation
   3. data acquisition system (DAS)
   4. postpatient collimation

   a. Only 1, 2, and 3 are correct.
   b. Only 1 and 3 are correct.
   c. Only 2 and 4 are correct.
   d. Only 4 is correct.
   e. All are correct.

73. Which of the following are useful features of a high-pressure xenon detector array?

1. fast response time
2. no afterglow
3. high geometric efficiency
4. high intrinsic efficiency

a. Only 1, 2, and 3 are correct.
b. Only 1 and 3 are correct.
c. Only 2 and 4 are correct.
d. Only 4 is correct.
e. All are correct.

74. Which of the following influences patient dose?

a. data acquisition system (DAS)
b. dose profile
c. postpatient collimator
d. prepatient collimator
e. section sensitivity profile

75. A multislice CT image is obtained at 130 kVp, 400 mA, 5 s. The resulting anode heat load is approximately

a. 200 joule (J).
b. 250 joule (J).
c. 300 joule (J).
d. 360 joule (J).
e. 420 joule (J).

76. Which of the following principally influences the section sensitivity profile?

a. prepatient collimator
b. postpatient collimator
c. data acquisition system (DAS)
d. detector response time
e. detector interspace

77. Filtration of the x-ray beam in a CT imager results in

a. reduced beam energy.
b. increased beam energy.
c. increased beam intensity.
d. fewer image artifacts.
e. reduced x-ray tube loading.

78. A beam-shaping filter is useful in CT imaging to

a. reduce patient dose.
b. equalize x-ray intensity at the detector array.
c. reduce imaging time.
d. reduce image artifacts.
e. allow smaller focal spot size.

79. The principal reason that high kVp is employed in CT imaging is reduced

a. scan time.
b. reconstruction time.
c. x-ray tube loading.
d. image noise.
e. image latitude.

80. The result of thin section imaging is
    a. a broader section sensitivity profile.
    b. better contrast resolution.
    c. reduced image noise.
    d. fewer partial volume artifacts.
    e. faster imaging time.

81. The ability to improve spatial resolution by use of a smaller focal spot in CT imaging results because of the
    a. accompanying higher beam filtration.
    b. ability to use higher kVp.
    c. ability to use higher rotor speed.
    d. focal spot collimation alignment.
    e. geometric projection, as in projection radiography.

82. Which of the following principally controls pixel size?
    1. prepatient collimation
    2. field of view (FOV)
    3. postpatient collimation
    4. matrix size

    a. Only 1, 2, and 3 are correct.
    b. Only 1 and 3 are correct.
    c. Only 2 and 4 are correct.
    d. Only 4 is correct.
    e. All are correct.

83. Slip ring technology allows
    1. no interscan delay.
    2. continuous data acquisition.
    3. continuous imaging.
    4. improved contrast resolution.

    a. Only 1, 2, and 3 are correct.
    b. Only 1 and 3 are correct.
    c. Only 2 and 4 are correct.
    d. Only 4 is correct.
    e. All are correct.

84. Which of the following is reduced by the use of high kVp during CT imaging?
    1. photoelectric absorption
    2. image dynamic range
    3. x-ray tube loading
    4. radiation intensity at the image receptor

    a. Only 1, 2, and 3 are correct.
    b. Only 1 and 3 are correct.
    c. Only 2 and 4 are correct.
    d. Only 4 is correct.
    e. All are correct.

85. The ideal dose profile should appear as

    a.
    b.
    c.
    d.
    e.

86. Reducing slice thickness in CT imaging results in

    a. better contrast resolution.
    b. better spatial resolution.
    c. faster image acquisition.
    d. less image noise.
    e. shorter image reconstruction.

87. Thinner CT section images result in

    a. better contrast resolution.
    b. faster image acquisition.
    c. higher patient dose.
    d. less image noise.
    e. shorter image reconstruction.

88. If section sensitivity profile exceeds dose profile, what suffers most?

    a. patient dose
    b. spatial resolution
    c. contrast resolution
    d. image noise
    e. image artifacts

89. Which of the following is reduced by using high kVp during CT imaging?

    a. Compton scatter
    b. image contrast
    c. image dynamic range
    d. x-ray tube loading
    e. x-ray tube life

90. Slip rings designed to transfer high voltage are generally

    a. air insulated.
    b. oil insulated.
    c. molybdenum rhodium alloy.
    d. tungsten molybdenum alloy.
    e. greased to reduce friction.

91. Slip rings designed to transfer detector signals are

    a. air insulated.
    b. oil insulated.
    c. molybdenum rhodium alloy.
    d. tungsten molybdenum alloy.
    e. greased to reduce friction.

92. **When slice thickness is reduced, patient dose increases because**
   a. imaging time is increased.
   b. kVp must be increased.
   c. dose profile is less square.
   d. section sensitivity profile is increased.
   e. mA is increased.

93. **A 40-cm field of view (FOV) is imaged using a 512 matrix, what is the pixel size?**
   a. 0.25 mm
   b. 0.4 mm
   c. 0.6 mm
   d. 0.8 mm
   e. 1.0 mm

94. **Which of the following would normally be found on the gantry of a fourth-generation CT imager?**
   1. x-ray source
   2. reconstruction computer
   3. detector array
   4. software filters

   a. Only 1, 2, and 3 are correct.
   b. Only 1 and 3 are correct.
   c. Only 2 and 4 are correct.
   d. Only 4 is correct.
   e. All are correct.

95. **Which of the following high-voltage generators is most likely to be mounted on the rotating gantry of a CT imager?**
   a. single phase half-wave rectified
   b. single phase full-wave rectified
   c. three phase 6 pulse
   d. three phase 12 pulse
   e. high frequency

96. **Which of the following does not require the high-voltage supply cables be wound or rewound each 360° rotation?**
   a. single phase half-wave rectified
   b. single phase full-wave rectified
   c. three phase 6 pulse
   d. three phase 12 pulse
   e. high frequency

97. **A 24-cm field of view (FOV) is imaged using a 512 matrix and 6 mm slice thickness, what is the approximate the voxel size?**
   a. 1 mm^3
   b. 2 mm^3
   c. 3 mm^3
   d. 4 mm^3
   e. 5 mm^3

98. **When comparing solid state radiation detectors with gas-filled detectors for CT imaging, solid state detectors**

    1. respond faster.
    2. have less afterglow.
    3. produce directly digitized signals.
    4. have higher intrinsic detection efficiency.

    a. Only 1, 2, and 3 are correct.
    b. Only 1 and 3 are correct.
    c. Only 2 and 4 are correct.
    d. Only 4 is correct.
    e. All are correct.

99. **The collimators in a CT imager**

    1. control scatter into the detector.
    2. change during exposure.
    3. determine one dimension of the voxel.
    4. determine one dimension of the pixel.

    a. Only 1, 2, and 3 are correct.
    b. Only 1 and 3 are correct.
    c. Only 2 and 4 are correct.
    d. Only 4 is correct.
    e. All are correct.

100. **The detectors in a CT scanner may consist of**

    1. xenon gas ionization chambers.
    2. sodium iodide/photodiodes.
    3. bismuth germinate/photodiodes.
    4. cadmium tungstate/photodiodes.

    a. Only 1, 2, and 3 are correct.
    b. Only 1 and 3 are correct.
    c. Only 2 and 4 are correct.
    d. Only 4 is correct.
    e. All are correct.

101. **The use of high kVp for CT imaging results in**

    a. wider dynamic range of the image.
    b. higher image contrast.
    c. faster image time.
    d. fewer image artifacts.
    e. increased x-ray tube loading.

Image Reconstruction

- Image reconstruction involves filtered back projection, resulting in a digital matrix, which can be postprocessed for additional image analysis.

- The object of image reconstruction from projections is to compute and assign a computed tomography (CT) number to each pixel.

- Computed tomography imaging involves data acquisition, image reconstruction, and image display.

- Between data acquisition and image reconstruction is **preprocessing**—reformatting and convolution.

- Following image display is postprocessing, recording, and archiving.

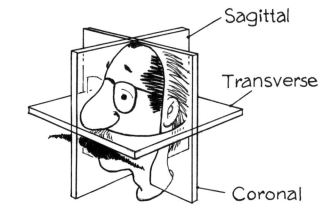

THE CT COMPUTER

- The CT computer must have exceptional capacity to manipulate the extensive data obtained.

- A CT computer consists of four principal components—an input device, a CPU, an output device, and memory.

- Input/output (I/O) devices are ancillary pieces of computer hardware designed to place raw data into a computer and receive processed data from the computer.

input devices :
- Keyboard
- disk

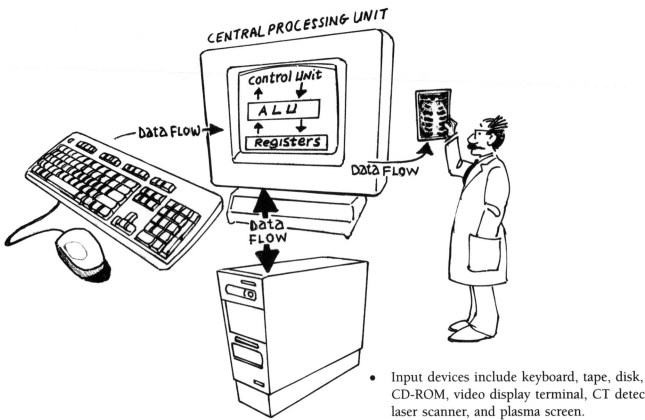

CENTRAL PROCESSING UNIT

control Unit

A L U

Registers

Data Flow

Data Flow

Data FLOW

output devices :
- CRT
- printer
- magnetic tape
- magnetic disk
- optical disk

- Input devices include keyboard, tape, disk, CD-ROM, video display terminal, CT detector, laser scanner, and plasma screen.

- Output devices include video display terminal, laser camera, dry image processor, printer, and image transmitter.

- **Hard copy** refers to an image on film or printed.

- **Soft copy** means the image is displayed on a cathode ray tube (CRT), flat panel display, or stored on magnetic or optical disks.

- The brains of a computer are in the central processing unit (CPU), which contains the microprocessor, the control unit, and primary memory.

- The microprocessor is the "computer on a chip," or wafer, of silicon fabricated into many diodes and transistors.

- The control unit interprets instructions, sequences tasks, and generally runs computer functions.

- RAM, ROM, or WORM are the three principal types of solid state memory—Random Access Memory, Read Only Memory, and Write One Read Many times memory.

- Look up tables (LUT) are software components.

- Primary memory exists as read only memory (ROM) or random access memory (RAM) to store data as it is used in computations.

- Primary memory may be on the CPU or on an additional circuit board.

- Primary memory is solid state, made of silicon (semiconductor) technology, and very fast but limited in size.

- Secondary memory is required when primary memory is insufficient and when data needs to be transferred to another location.

- Secondary memory is useful for bulk storage of information, such as images.

- Secondary memory can be on-line as with magnetic hard drive disks or off-line as with magnetic tape and magnetic or optical disks.

- The **analog-to-digital converter (ADC)** is a special type of computer that converts the analog signal from each CT detector to a digital form for computer manipulation.

- An **array processor** is a special type of computer that is designed to do only a special task, such as image reconstruction, and it does that task very fast.

- The **software** of a computer is the collection of programs written in computer language to implement the many tasks of a computer.

- There are two general types of software—**operating systems** and **application programs**.

- Operating systems such as Microsoft DOS, Microsoft Windows, and UNIX manages the computer hardware.

- Application programs are written in a higher level language.

- Application programs for CT include the algorithms for image reconstruction and programs for postprocessing analysis.

- The CT computer must have the capacity to solve a large number of equations simultaneously.

- To produce a 512 x 512 matrix, 512^2 or 262,144 equations must be solved simultaneously.

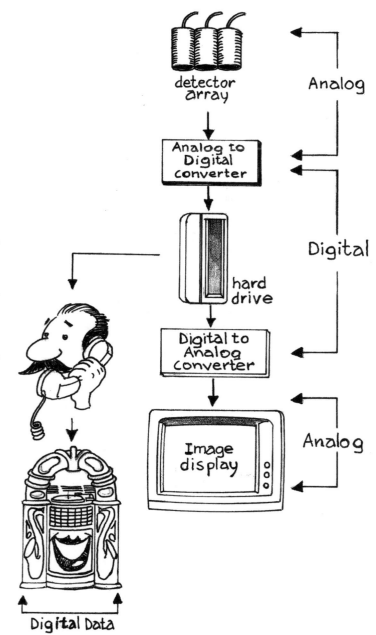

if the image matrix is	then	the number of simultaneous equations is
2 X 2		4
4 x 4		16
128 x 128		16,384
256 x 256		65,536
512 x 512		262,144
1024 x 1024		1,048,576

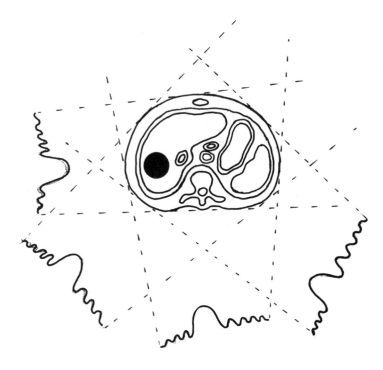

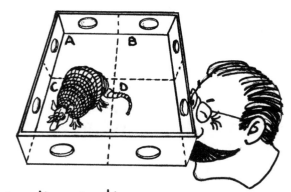

backprojection
reconstruction from
image profile

- The laboratory environment should be controlled to less than 30% relative humidity and below 20°C (70°F) to ensure best computer operation.

- The time from the end of imaging (end of data collection) to image appearance is the **reconstruction time.**

- Reconstruction times of 1 s and less are common.

- Most of the action of a CT computer is accomplished with multiple microprocessors.

- Most image reconstruction is done with an **array processor.**

- The array processor is designed to perform many specific calculations very quickly, but can do nothing else.

BACK PROJECTION

- The analog image projection recorded by each detector element is received and transferred by the data acquisition system (DAS) to the ADC so it becomes a digital image projection.

- Each digital image projection acquired by each detector during a CT examination is stored in the computer memory.

- Computed tomography images are reconstructed from these image projections by convoluted back projection.

- The image is reconstructed with simultaneous filtered back projection of all the image projections.

- Reconstruction algorithms are a set of well-defined computer software steps designed to produce a specific output (image) from a given input (signal profiles).

- Four reconstruction algorithms have been applied to CT—Fourier transformation, analytic, iterative, and back projection.

- Back projection with a convolution filter —filtered back projection—is most widely applied in CT.

- Volume and surface rendered images are produced with different convolution filters.

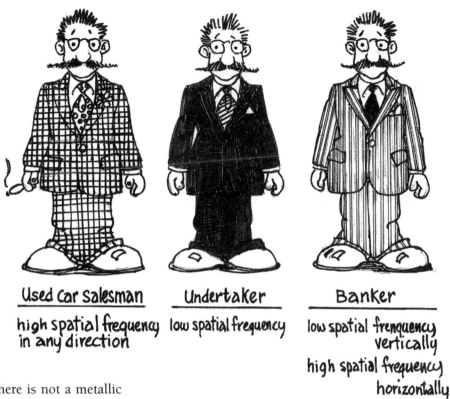

Used Car salesman
high spatial frequency in any direction

Undertaker
low spatial frequency

Banker
low spatial frenquency vertically
high spatial frequency horizontally

- The word **filter** as used here is not a metallic filter of Al or Cu placed in an x-ray beam to reduce low energy x-rays.

- Filter, or more correctly, **convolution filter**, refers to a mathematical manipulation of the data designed to change the appearance of the image.

- A convolution filter—sometimes called a **kernel**—is a mathematics process applied to an image projection before back projection.

- Convolution filters are also called **reconstruction algorithms**.

- A high-frequency convolution filter suppresses high-frequency signals, causing the image to have a smooth appearance and possible improvement in contrast resolution.

- Back projection results in a blurred image because x-ray attenuation is not uniform over the entire path length.

- The convolution filter is applied to the image projections prior to reconstruction and the result is a sharper image.

- A low-frequency convolution filter suppresses low-frequency signals, resulting in edge enhancement and possible improvement in spatial resolution.

Q: what is the limiting spatial
   frequency if the pixel size is 0.5mm?

A: One line pair = a 0.5mm line + 0.5mm interspace.
   spatial frequency = 0.5 + 0.5 = 1.0 lp/mm

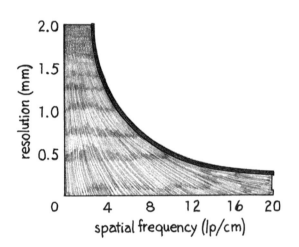

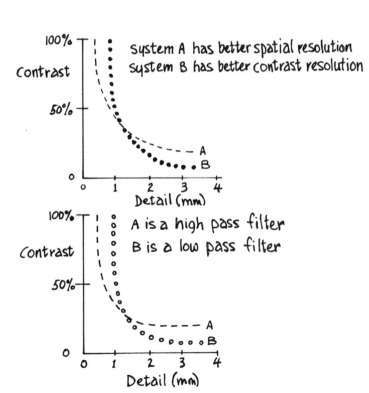

System A has better spatial resolution
System B has better contrast resolution

A is a high pass filter
B is a low pass filter

- Most CT imagers have in excess of 20 convolution filters available that are operator selectable.

- Image projections from all angles are overlapped.

- Projection angulation results in image blur, which can be accommodated by **convolution filters**.

- There are many types of convolution filters—some enhance contrast resolution, some enhance spatial resolution.

- Spatial frequency relates how rapidly subject contrast changes.

- A bone-soft tissue interface represents high-spatial frequency (small object, high contrast).

- Gray matter-white matter of brain represents low-spatial frequency (large object, low contrast).

- The spatial frequencies of various tissues are enhanced or suppressed by using appropriate convolution filters.

- High-pass convolution filters enhance high-spatial frequencies and suppress low-spatial frequencies.

- High-pass convolution filters are used for imaging of bone, inner ear, etc.

- High-pass convolution filters (bone algorithms) result in images with enhanced edges, short scale of contrast, and more noise.

- Low-pass convolution filters enhance low-spatial frequencies and suppress high-spatial frequencies.

- Low-pass convolution filters are used for imaging soft tissue such as brain, liver, etc.

- Low-pass convolution filters (smoothing algorithms) appear less noisy with long scale of contrast.

- Image reconstruction time is 1 s or less and is determined by ADC rate, CPU clock speed, amount of data collected, and convolution filter chosen.

IMAGE DISPLAY

- All CT images are digital and formatted as a matrix.

- A matrix is an orderly array of cells fashioned in rows and columns.

- Current CT imagers produce 512×512 images and 1024×1024 is available on many.

- A 1024×1024 image is reconstructed from $1024^2 = 1,048,576$ simultaneous equations into $1,048,576$ matrix cells.

- A larger matrix size results in improved spatial resolution.

- A larger matrix size requires longer reconstruction time.

- Each matrix cell is a *pi*cture *el*ement (pixel).

- Each pixel is a two-dimensional representation of a *vo*lume *el*ement (voxel).

- Voxel size is the product of pixel size and section thickness.

- The diameter of the reconstructed image is the **field of view (FOV)**.

- When FOV is increased and matrix size is constant, pixel size increases and spatial resolution is reduced.

- Either smaller FOV or larger matrix size results in smaller pixel size.

- When FOV is constant and matrix size increased, pixel size is reduced and spatial resolution improved.

- In general, pixel size is the limiting spatial resolution of a CT imager.

- Small pixel images have improved spatial resolution and contain high-frequency information.

- Large pixel images have reduced spatial resolution and contain more low-frequency information.

- Matrix size describes the number of pixels in an image.

- Spatial resolution is determined by matrix size and FOV.

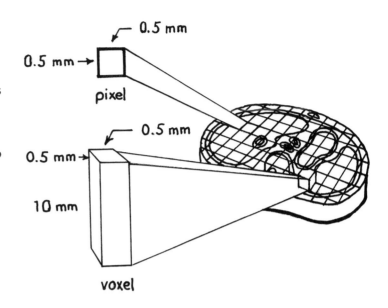

$$\text{pixel size} = \frac{FOV}{matrix}$$

Q: What is the pixel size if the FOV is 20 cm with a 512^2 matrix?

A: $\text{pixel size} = \dfrac{200\,mm}{512} = 0.39\ mm$

Matrix Size	FOV	Pixel Size
512 × 512	12 cm	0.23 mm
512 × 512	30 cm	0.59 mm
1024 × 1024	12 cm	0.12 mm
1024 × 1024	30 cm	0.29 mm

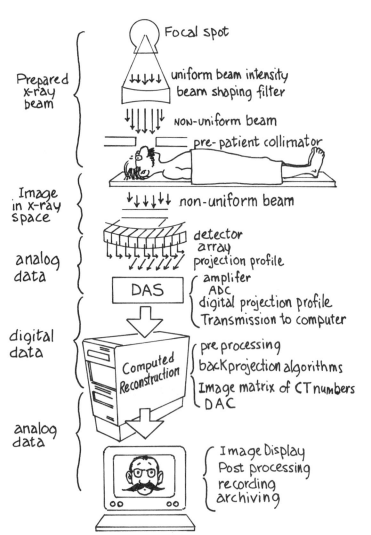

- Larger matrix size, for example 1024^2 instead of 512^2, results in smaller pixels and better spatial resolution.

- Smaller matrix size is useful for pediatric imaging.

- Smaller matrix size is useful for biopsy localization.

- The normal scanned FOV is approximately 20 cm for head or pediatric body, 35 cm for body, and 48 cm for large body.

- Localizer images are used to plan extent of anatomy to be imaged.

- Localizer images are an example of digital radiographic images.

- Computed tomography vendors identify localizer images by various names . . . Scoutview, Pilotscan, Topogram, and Surview.

- Localizer images are made with the x-ray beam on continuously while the patient couch moves through the beam.

- Localizer images may be AP, PA, or lateral.

- The display FOV can be equal to or less than the scanned field of view (SFOV).

- Pixel size is the quotient of FOV by matrix size.

- There is a subtle difference between SFOV and displayed field of view (DFOV).

- Scanned field of view is usually set to cover the anatomic part—head, body, large body.

- Displayed field of view is usually employed as a postprocessing tool to provide a magnified image of a part of the SFOV.

- Magnification using original image projections—**target zoom**—results in improvement in spatial resolution.

- Magnification resulting from pixel enlargement—**photo zoom**—is easier and faster but the image has less spatial resolution than the original.

- Postprocessing includes image pan and zoom; histogram analysis; distance and area analysis; annotation; multi-image display; quantitative CT; windowing; contrast control and reversal; image rotation; and collage and coronal, sagittal, and oblique reconstruction, smoothing, and enhancement.

- Postprocessing does not result in additional information, just the same or less information presented differently.

CT NUMBERS

- The solution of the simultaneous equations by filtered back projection results in a numerical value (CT number) for each pixel.

- The CT number is directly related to the x-ray linear attenuation coefficient (μ) for the tissue in that voxel.

- The standard scale of CT numbers is the Hounsfield scale of Hounsfield units (HU)—not to be confused with heat units.

- According to the Hounsfield scale dense bone = 1000 HU, water = 0 HU, and air = −1000 HU.

- One HU = 0.1% difference between μ of tissue compared to μ of water.

- Pixel brightness is proportional to HU—high HU is bright, low HU dark.

- The Hounsfield scale ranges from −1000 to +1000 and some imagers have CT number scale from −2000 to +6000.

- The video monitor can display perhaps 256 shades of gray but the eye can detect only approximately 20.

- The range of CT numbers displayed is the **window width (WW).**

- The central value of the WW is the window level (WL).

- Reducing WW increases contrast.

- The WL selects the CT number at the center of the displayed gray scale.

- Window width (WW) and level (WL) allow the entire CT or HU number scale to be visualized.

$$CT\ number = k\left(\frac{\mu_t - \mu_w}{\mu_w}\right)$$

$$when\ k = 1000,\ CT\ number = HU$$

Tissue	HU (at 125 kVp)	μ
Dense bone	1000	0.460
Muscle	50	0.231
White matter	45	0.187
Gray matter	40	0.184
Blood	20	0.182
Cerebrospinal fluid	15	0.181
Water	0	0.180
Fat	−100	0.162
Lungs	−200	0.094
Air	−1000	0.0003

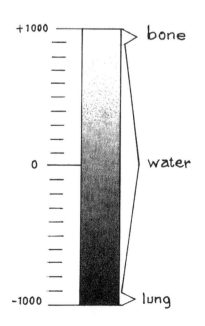

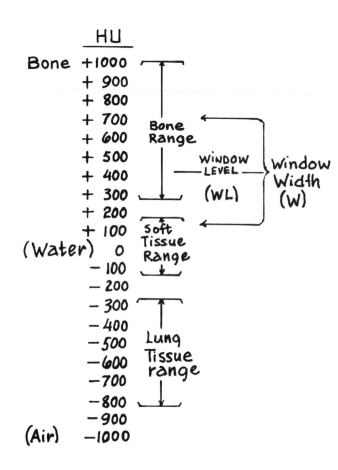

HU

Bone	+1000	
	+ 900	
	+ 800	
	+ 700	Bone Range
	+ 600	
	+ 500	
	+ 400	WINDOW LEVEL (WL)
	+ 300	
	+ 200	
	+ 100	Soft Tissue Range
(Water)	0	
	− 100	
	− 200	
	− 300	
	− 400	
	− 500	Lung Tissue range
	− 600	
	− 700	
	− 800	
	− 900	
(Air)	−1000	

Window Width (W)

Typical WW and WL viewing

	WW	WL
Brain : posterior fossa	100	40
brain	80	40
Chest : soft tissue	400	40
lung	1500	-400
Abdomen	400	50
C-spine : soft Tissue	500	60
bone	1600	300
T-spine : soft tissue	500	60
bone	1600	300
Orbit : Soft tissue	400	30
brain	100	40
bone	3000	500
Bone : Temporal	3000	500
Spine	1600	300

- Wide WW is used for bone imaging, narrow WW for soft tissue.

- Windowing refers to the manipulation of WL and WW to optimize image contrast.

- A wide WW results in a gray image—long gray scale, low contrast.

- A narrow WW results in a black/white image—short gray scale, high contrast.

- Window level is the center of WW.

- A CT image is optimized for that tissue having the same CT number as the WL.

POSTPROCESSING

- Most widely applied multiplanar reconstruction (MPR) algorithms result in maximum intensity projection (MIP) and shaded-surface display (SSD).

- Multiplanar reconstruction produces coronal and sagittal images from stacked transverse images.

- Quantitative CT (QCT) compares vertebral bone CT numbers with a standard phantom imaged simultaneously to assay bone mineralization.

MAXIMUM INTENSITY PROJECTION (MIP)

- Multiple MIP images reconstructed at different angles and viewed in rotation may be required to separate superimposed vessels.

- Maximum intensity projection was first employed in MRI.

- Maximum intensity projection is the basis for computed tomography angiography (CTA).

- To create the proper image plane, the technologist must have a good foundation in anatomy, especially vascular anatomy.

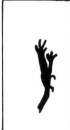

Projected image

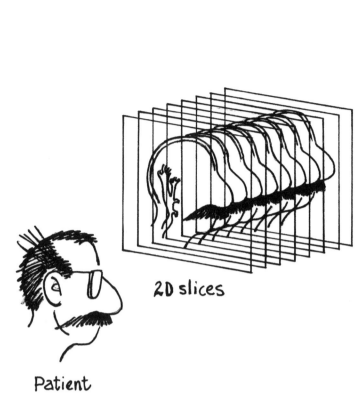

2D slices

Patient

- Maximum intensity projection selects voxels along a row or column in a volume of interest (VOI) with the highest CT number—or a specified range of CT number—for display.

- Bones usually have higher CT number than contrast-filled vessels and must be software excluded.

- Multiple overlapping reconstruction reduces the "beading" artifact sometimes seen in MIP.

- Along any row or column, the voxel with the highest CT number is displayed.

- Contrast-enhanced voxels are displayed in preference to soft tissue voxels.

- Maximum intensity projection images do not provide depth information.

- Maximum intensity projection images are volume-rendered images.

- Shaded surface images are surface-rendered images.

- The width of the region of interest (ROI) should be as small as possible to reduce background noise in the presence of contrast-filled vessels.

CT post processing features
 – change contrast scale
 – ROI for QCT
 – linear measurement
 – volume measurement
 – surface rendering
 – volume rendering
 – CT angiography

Chapter 4 Practice Questions

1. The analytical technique used to reconstruct most CT images is
   a. filtered back projection.
   b. Fourier transformation.
   c. iterative reconstruction.
   d. repetitive back projection.
   e. two-dimensional Fourier transformation.

2. The proper sequence for producing a CT image is
   a. data acquisition, image postprocessing, image reconstruction.
   b. data acquisition, image reconstruction, image postprocessing.
   c. image postprocessing, data acquisition, image reconstruction.
   d. image reconstruction, data acquisition, image postprocessing.
   e. image reconstruction, image postprocessing, data acquisition.

3. Usually, images are postprocessed to
   a. speed imaging time.
   b. improve contrast resolution.
   c. provide additional image analysis.
   d. reduce the x-ray tube load.
   e. provide multiple slices.

4. Which of the following would be included in the four principal components of the CT computer?
   1. a central processing unit (CPU)
   2. an input device
   3. memory
   4. an output device

   a. Only 1, 2, and 3 are correct.
   b. Only 1 and 3 are correct.
   c. Only 2 and 4 are correct.
   d. Only 4 is correct.
   e. All are correct.

5. Which of the following is an input device for use with the CT imager?
   a. cathode ray tube (CRT)
   b. keyboard
   c. magnetic disk
   d. optical disk
   e. video display terminal

6. What is the approximate limiting spatial frequency of a CT image with 12-cm FOV reconstructed with a 512 matrix?
   a. 1 lp/cm
   b. 3 lp/cm
   c. 5 lp/cm
   d. 10 lp/cm
   e. 20 lp/cm

7. **Which of the following is an output device used in CT imaging?**

    a. a laser scanner
    b. a plasma screen
    c. an electronic mouse
    d. cathode ray tube (CRT)
    e. keyboard

8. **To reconstruct a CT image with a 1024 × 1024 matrix, approximately how many equations must be solved simultaneously?**

    a. 100
    b. 1000
    c. 10,000
    d. 100,000
    e. 1,000,000

9. **Which of the following would be a hard copy CT image?**

    a. laser film
    b. magnetic disk
    c. magnetic tape
    d. optical disk
    e. video monitor screen

10. **Field of view (FOV) refers to the**

    a. area of the patient aperture.
    b. area of the reconstructed image.
    c. diameter of the patient aperture.
    d. diameter of the reconstructed image.
    e. total number of picture elements.

11. **The central processing unit (CPU) of a CT computer contains**

    a. a microprocessor.
    b. an optical disk.
    c. the back projector.
    d. the image reconstructor.
    e. the video display terminal.

12. **Which of the following is the correct formula for the Hounsfield Unit (HU)?**

    a. $500\left(\dfrac{\mu_t - \mu_w}{\mu_w}\right)$

    b. $500\left(\dfrac{\mu_w - \mu_t}{\mu_w}\right)$

    c. $1000\left(\dfrac{\mu_t - \mu_w}{\mu_w}\right)$

    d. $1000\left(\dfrac{\mu_w - \mu_t}{\mu_w}\right)$

    e. $k\left(\dfrac{\mu_w - \mu_t}{\mu_w}\right)$

13. **The central processing unit (CPU) of a CT imager is**
    a. an optical disk.
    b. primary memory.
    c. the back projector.
    d. the image reconstructor.
    e. the video display terminal.

14. **Which of the following is a useful postprocessing maneuver?**
    1. pan and zoom
    2. histogram analysis
    3. region of interest (ROI)
    4. windowing

    a. Only 1, 2, and 3 are correct.
    b. Only 1 and 3 are correct.
    c. Only 2 and 4 are correct.
    d. Only 4 is correct.
    e. All are correct.

15. **The control unit of the central processing unit (CPU) is responsible principally for**
    a. image postprocessing.
    b. image reconstruction.
    c. random access memory (RAM).
    d. read-only memory (ROM).
    e. running functions.

16. **RAM, ROM, and WORM are all types of**
    a. computer algorithms.
    b. solid state memory.
    c. reconstruction algorithms.
    d. postprocessing algorithms.
    e. image templates.

17. **Primary memory consists of**
    1. random access memory (RAM).
    2. read-only memory (ROM).
    3. reconstruction algorithms.
    4. lookup tables (LUT).

    a. Only 1, 2, and 3 are correct.
    b. Only 1 and 3 are correct.
    c. Only 2 and 4 are correct.
    d. Only 4 is correct.
    e. All are correct.

18. **Maximum intensity projection images are termed**
    a. leveled images.
    b. region of interest (ROI) images.
    c. surface rendered images.
    d. volume rendered images.
    e. windowed images.

19. LUT employed in the CT imager stands for

    a. light utility tables.
    b. light utility template.
    c. long of a template.
    d. lookup tables
    e. lookup templates.

20. The analog-to-digital converter (ADC) in a CT imager is

    a. a special type of dedicated computer.
    b. part of the rotating gantry.
    c. part of the stationary gantry.
    d. the site of image postprocessing.
    e. the site of image reconstruction.

21. Which of the following would be an example of multiplanar reconstruction?

    a. displayed field of view (DFOV)
    b. Hounsfield units (HU)
    c. quantitative CT (QCT)
    d. region of interest (ROI)
    e. shaded surface display (SSD)

22. Which of the following could be identified as a special type of computer used in CT imaging?

    1. analog-to-digital converter (ADC)
    2. central processing unit (CPU)
    3. array processor
    4. lookup tables (LUT)

    a. Only 1, 2, and 3 are correct.
    b. Only 1 and 3 are correct.
    c. Only 2 and 4 are correct.
    d. Only 4 is correct.
    e. All are correct.

23. Although a video monitor can display perhaps an 8 bit contrast level (256 shades of gray), the human eye can distinguish only approximately

    a. 5 shades of gray.
    b. 10 shades of gray.
    c. 20 shades of gray.
    d. 50 shades of gray.
    e. 100 shades of gray.

24. Which of the following would be identified as software used in a CT imager?

    a. analog-to-digital converter (ADC)
    b. array processor
    c. central processing unit (CPU)
    d. random access memory (RAM)
    e. reconstruction algorithm

25. The formula for computing the value of the CT number is based on the
    a. electron density of water.
    b. linear attenuation coefficient for water.
    c. mass attenuation coefficient for water.
    d. mass density of water.
    e. molecular composition of water.

26. Which of the following best represents a high-frequency anatomic object?
    a. bone-lung
    b. cartilage-muscle
    c. gray matter-white matter
    d. liver-spleen
    e. muscle-fat

27. The principal application of quantitative CT (QCT) is
    a. bone mineral assay.
    b. Computed tomography angiography (CTA).
    c. displayed field of view (FOV).
    d. histographic analysis.
    e. region of interest (ROI) display.

28. Reconstruction algorithms are an example of
    a. an analog-to-digital converter (ADC).
    b. an application program.
    c. an array processor.
    d. primary memory.
    e. secondary memory.

29. Which of the following window levels/window widths would be most appropriate for imaging lung?
    a. WW 100 WL 40
    b. WW 400 WL 50
    c. WW 1500 WL 300
    d. WW 1500 WL −400
    e. WW 3000 WL −800

30. Routine image reconstruction times are
    a. ≤1 second.
    b. 2−4 seconds.
    c. 3−7 seconds.
    d. 5−10 seconds.
    e. >10 seconds.

31. Most image reconstruction is done with which part of a CT imager?
    a. analog-to-digital (ADC)
    b. lookup tables (LUT)
    c. random access memory (RAM)
    d. array processor
    e. back projector

32. The CT number for water when expressed as a Houndsfield unit (HU) has a value of

    a. −1000.
    b. −500.
    c. 0.
    d. +500.
    e. +1000.

33. Reconstruction algorithms are

    a. a convolution filter.
    b. computer software.
    c. lookup tables (LUT).
    d. the array processor.
    e. the kernel.

34. A localizer image differs from a CT image because

    a. image postprocessing is required.
    b. image reformation is required.
    c. it appears as a digital radiograph.
    d. the patient moves continuously while the x-ray beam is pulsed.
    e. the patient moves step-by-step while the x-ray beam is on continuously.

35. Convolution filters are applied in CT imaging to

    a. change the appearance of the image.
    b. process an image.
    c. reconstruct multiple images simultaneously.
    d. reconstruct the image.
    e. reduce patient dose.

36. Which of the following window levels/window widths would be most appropriate for imaging soft tissue?

    a. WW 100 WL 40
    b. WW 400 WL 50
    c. WW 1500 WL 300
    d. WW 1500 WL −400
    e. WW 3000 WL −800

37. A low-frequency convolution filter will normally produce a/an

    a. smooth appearing image with improved contrast resolution.
    b. smooth appearing image with improved spatial resolution.
    c. sharper appearing image with improved contrast resolution.
    d. sharper appearing image with improved spatial resolution.
    e. image with improved contrast and spatial resolution.

38. Which of the following gives the appearance of a smoother image with less noise?

    a. low-frequency convolution filter
    b. high-frequency convolution filter
    c. analog lookup table
    d. digital lookup table
    e. data acquisition system (DAS)

39. Which of the following will be identified as a CT reconstruction algorithm?

   1. kernel
   2. lookup table (LUT)
   3. convolution filter
   4. Fourier transformation

   a. Only 1, 2, and 3 are correct.
   b. Only 1 and 3 are correct.
   c. Only 2 and 4 are correct.
   d. Only 4 is correct.
   e. All are correct.

40. When the CT number for bone is expressed as a Houndsfield unit (HU), its value is approximately

   a. -1000.
   b. -500.
   c. 0.
   d. $+500$.
   e. $+1000$.

41. Which of the following best represents a low-frequency anatomic object?

   a. bone-muscle
   b. bone-lung
   c. brain-cranium
   d. eye-orbit
   e. liver-spleen

42. Which of the following would be considered a software component of a CT imager?

   1. operating system
   2. lookup tables (LUT)
   3. application programs
   4. reconstruction algorithms

   a. Only 1, 2, and 3 are correct.
   b. Only 1 and 3 are correct.
   c. Only 2 and 4 are correct.
   d. Only 4 is correct.
   e. All are correct.

43. The value of the CT number is related principally to

   a. effective atomic number
   b. hydrogen concentration.
   c. mass density.
   d. optical density.
   e. the x-ray linear attenuation coefficient.

44. A low-pass convolution filter would most likely be used to image

   a. bone-lung.
   b. gray matter-white matter.
   c. bone-muscle.
   d. brain-cranium.
   e. eye-orbit.

45. Which of the following are characteristics of an image produced with a low-pass convolution filter?

    1. smooth appearance
    2. less noise
    3. long contrast scale
    4. better contrast resolution

    a. Only 1, 2, and 3 are correct.
    b. Only 1 and 3 are correct.
    c. Only 2 and 4 are correct.
    d. Only 4 is correct.
    e. All are correct.

46. An image produced with a high-pass convolution filter would likely appear

    1. noisy.
    2. with short contrast scale.
    3. with improved spatial resolution.
    4. with better contrast resolution.

    a. Only 1, 2, and 3 are correct.
    b. Only 1 and 3 are correct.
    c. Only 2 and 4 are correct.
    d. Only 4 is correct.
    e. All are correct.

47. When viewing a CT image, the term window level refers to the

    a. central CT number of the window width.
    b. lowest CT number of the window width.
    c. highest CT number of the window width.
    d. contrast range reconstructed.
    e. contrast range displayed.

48. 0.3 mm lines separated by 0.3 mm interspaces create what approximate spatial frequency?

    a. 3 lp/cm
    b. 6 lp/cm
    c. 10 lp/cm
    d. 14 lp/cm
    e. 17 lp/cm

49. Which of the following results in improved spatial resolution?

    a. magnification zoom
    b. photographic zoom
    c. reduced displayed field of view (DFOV)
    d. reduced scanned field of view (SFOV)
    e. target zoom

50. What is the limiting spatial frequency for a CT image with a pixel size of 0.4 mm?

    a. 8 lp/cm
    b. 13 lp/cm
    c. 16 lp/cm
    d. 20 lp/cm
    e. 25 lp/cm

51. Which of the following is an input device for use with the CT scanner?
    a. cathode ray tube (CRT)
    b. magnetic disk
    c. optical disk
    d. plasma screen
    e. video display terminal

52. The principal image characteristic of computed tomography is
    a. contrast resolution.
    b. linearity.
    c. multiplonar reconstruction.
    d. noise.
    e. spatial resolution.

53. What is the approximate limiting spatial frequency of a 12-cm field of view (FOV) CT image with a 1024 × 1024 matrix?
    a. 5 lp/cm
    b. 10 lp/cm
    c. 15 lp/cm
    d. 25 lp/cm
    e. 40 lp/cm

54. Which of the following is likely to improve spatial resolution?
    1. reduced field of view (FOV)
    2. high-frequency convolution filter
    3. increased matrix size
    4. increased kVp

    a. Only 1, 2, and 3 are correct.
    b. Only 1 and 3 are correct.
    c. Only 2 and 4 are correct.
    d. Only 4 is correct.
    e. All are correct.

55. A 1024 × 1024 CT image contains approximately how many pixels?
    a. 100
    b. 1000
    c. 10,000
    d. 100,000
    e. 1,000,000

56. Which of the following is an output device used in CT imaging?
    a. laser scanner
    b. plasma screen
    c. electronic mouse
    d. keyboard
    e. optical disk

57. To reconstruct a CT image in a 512 × 512 matrix, approximately how many simultaneous equations are required?

    a. 5000
    b. 25,000
    c. 50,000
    d. 250,000
    e. 500,000

58. The principal advantage of a larger matrix size in a reconstructed CT image is

    a. ease of image processing.
    b. improved contrast resolution.
    c. improved spatial resolution.
    d. reduced noise.
    e. reduced patient dose.

59. The displayed field of view (DFOV) is

    a. a postprocessing maneuver to produce a magnified image.
    b. reduced when the postprocessing algorithm is limited.
    c. used when the data acquisition system (DAS) is limited.
    d. useful in suppressing high-frequency structures.
    e. useful in suppressing low-frequency structures.

60. Which of the following would be a soft copy CT image?

    a. laser film
    b. multiformat camera
    c. paper printer
    d. Polaroid image
    e. video display terminal

61. A 512 × 512 image matrix contains approximately how many pixels?

    a. 5000
    b. 25,000
    c. 50,000
    d. 250,000
    e. 500,000

62. Which of the following is most likely to limit the spatial resolution of a CT image?

    a. convolution filter
    b. data acquisition system (DAS)
    c. field of view (FOV)
    d. matrix size
    e. pixel size

63. When comparing a 512^2 matrix to a 1024^2 image matrix, the 1024^2 matrix

    a. contains an increased number of pixels determined by field of view (FOV).
    b. contains four times as many pixels.
    c. contains twice the number of pixels.
    d. will have better contrast resolution.
    e. will have less image noise.

64. Another term for convolution filter is

 a. back projection.
 b. Fourier transformation.
 c. kernel.
 d. lookup table (LUT).
 e. shaped metallic insert.

65. The displayed field of view (DFOV)

 a. can be equal to or less than the scanned field of view (SFOV).
 b. can be equal to or more than the scanned field of view (SFOV).
 c. is determined by area of the patient aperture.
 d. is determined by diameter of the patient aperture.
 e. must be equal to the scanned field of view (SFOV).

66. Pixel size is computed by

 a. field of view (FOV) divided by matrix size.
 b. field of view (FOV) squared multiplied by matrix size.
 c. field of view (FOV) squared divided by matrix size.
 d. field of view (FOV) multiplied by matrix size.
 e. matrix size divided by field of view (FOV).

67. A principal disadvantage of a larger CT image matrix is

 a. compromised postprocessing.
 b. artifacts.
 c. longer reconstruction time.
 d. reduced contrast resolution.
 e. reduced spatial resolution.

68. What is the limiting spatial frequency for a CT image with a pixel size of 1 mm?

 a. 5 lp/cm
 b. 8 lp/cm
 c. 12 lp/cm
 d. 16 lp/cm
 e. 20 lp/cm

69. The central processing unit (CPU) contains which of the following components?

 1. microprocessor
 2. control unit
 3. primary memory
 4. secondary memory

 a. Only 1, 2, and 3 are correct.
 b. Only 1 and 3 are correct.
 c. Only 2 and 4 are correct.
 d. Only 4 is correct.
 e. All are correct.

70. **The value of a CT number is directly related to**
    a. Compton interaction.
    b. photoelectric interaction.
    c. the tissue component of that voxel.
    d. the tissues in the displayed field of view (DFOV).
    e. the tissues in the scanned field of view (SFOV).

71. **A high-pass convolution filter would most likely be used to image**
    a. bone-lung.
    b. cartilage-muscle.
    c. gray matter-white matter.
    d. liver-spleen.
    e. muscle-fat.

72. **Which of the following would be identified as software used in a CT imager?**
    a. analog-to-digital converter (ADC)
    b. application programs
    c. array processor
    d. central processing unit (CPU)
    e. random access memory (RAM)

73. **When CT numbers are expressed as Houndsfield units (HU), the value of air is**
    a. −1000.
    b. −500.
    c. 0.
    d. +500.
    e. +1000.

74. **Which of the following is the normal sequence of CT imaging?**
    a. detector array–DAS–ADC–array processor
    b. DAS–ADC–array processor–detector array
    c. ADC–detector array–DAS–array processor
    d. array processor–detector array–ADC–DAS
    e. ADC–DAS–detector array–array processor

75. **Reduction of image blur in reconstructed CT images is accomplished with**
    a. analog-to-digital converter (ADC).
    b. convolution filters.
    c. digital-to-analog converter.
    d. Fourier transformation.
    e. iterated reconstruction.

76. **Concerning the numerical value of a pixel,**
    a. higher is brighter.
    b. higher is more contrast.
    c. higher is more dense.
    d. lower is brighter.
    e. lower is more dense.

77. **Which of the following would be identified as software used in a CT imager?**

    a. analog-to-digital converter (ADC)
    b. array processor
    c. central processing unit (CPU)
    d. lookup tables (LUT)
    e. random access memory (RAM)

78. **When viewing a CT image, the term window width (WW) refers to the**

    a. contrast range in CT number.
    b. lowest CT number that appears black.
    c. highest CT number that appears white.
    d. number shades of gray reconstructed.
    e. number of shades of gray viewed.

79. **0.2 mm lines separated by 0.2 mm interspaces create what spatial frequency?**

    a. 10 lp/cm
    b. 20 lp/cm
    c. 25 lp/cm
    d. 40 lp/cm
    e. 50 lp/cm

80. **One method of increasing the contrast of a CT image is to**

    a. increase kVp.
    b. increase mA.
    c. increase scan time.
    d. reduce the window width (WW).
    e. reduce the window level (WL).

81. **The central processing unit (CPU) of a CT computer contains**

    a. an optical disk.
    b. the back projector.
    c. the control unit.
    d. the image reconstructor.
    e. the video display terminal.

82. **Which of the following would be an example of multiplanar reconstruction (MPR)?**

    a. displayed field of view (DFOV)
    b. Hounsfield units (HU)
    c. maximum intensity projection (MIP)
    d. quantitative CT (QCT)
    e. region of interest (ROI)

83. **An array processor as employed in CT imaging is**

    a. a special type of dedicated computer.
    b. part of the rotating gantry.
    c. part of the stationary gantry.
    d. the site of image postprocessing.
    e. the site of image reconstruction.

84. The operating system of the CT imager controls the

    a. computer hardware.
    b. image postprocessing.
    c. image reconstruction.
    d. imaging sequence.
    e. pre- and postprocessing collimation.

85. Computed tomography angiography (CTA) is possible because of

    a. displayed field of view (DFOV).
    b. maximum intensity projection (MIP).
    c. quantitative CT (QCT).
    d. shaded-surface display.
    e. shaded-volume display.

86. Which of the following would be classified as postprocessing of a CT image?

    1. region of interest (ROI)
    2. surface rendering
    3. maximum intensity projection
    4. windowing

    a. Only 1, 2, and 3 are correct.
    b. Only 1 and 3 are correct.
    c. Only 2 and 4 are correct.
    d. Only 4 is correct.
    e. All are correct.

87. Which of the following would **not** be identified as primary memory?

    a. DRAM
    b. LUT
    c. RAM
    d. ROM
    e. WORM

88. Which of the following window levels/window widths would be most appropriate for imaging brain?

    a. WW 100 WL 40
    b. WW 400 WL 50
    c. WW 1500 WL 300
    d. WW 1500 WL 400
    e. WW 3000 WL 500

89. Image reconstruction time is defined as that from

    a. patient positioning to patient dismissal.
    b. patient positioning to start of scanning.
    c. start of scanning to end of scanning.
    d. end of scanning to image appearance.
    e. start of scanning to image appearance.

90. A high-frequency convolution filter will normally produce a/an
    a. smooth appearing image with improved contrast resolution.
    b. smooth appearing image with improved spatial resolution.
    c. sharper appearing image with improved contrast resolution.
    d. sharper appearing image with improved spatial resolution.
    e. image with improved contrast and spatial resolution.

91. Which of the following window levels/window widths would be most appropriate for imaging bone?
    a. WW 100 WL 40
    b. WW 400 WL 50
    c. WW 1500 WL 300
    d. WW 1500 WL 400
    e. WW 3000 WL 500

92. How many bits are required for each CT image if the matrix size is 512 and the CT number range is 4096?
    a. 512×4096
    b. $512 \times 512 \times 12$
    c. $512 \times 512 \times 512$
    d. $512 \times 512 \times 2048$
    e. $512 \times 512 \times 4096$

93. A single 512 x 512 image with 16 bit dynamic range requires how much storage?
    a. 0.5 MB
    b. 1.1 MB
    c. 2.2 MB
    d. 4.2 MB
    e. 10.2 MB

94. The fundamental measurement made by a CT imager is the
    a. sorting of CT numbers.
    b. determination of gray scale.
    c. number of pixels.
    d. relative absorption of x-rays.
    e. number of voxels.

95. In a CT imager
    1. the x-ray beam is usually collimated at the tube and at the detectors.
    2. a pixel refers to a picture element making up the image matrix.
    3. an 80 x 80 matrix contains 6400 pixels.
    4. a voxel is a picture element located at the patient's vocal cord.

    a. Only 1, 2, and 3 are correct.
    b. Only 1 and 3 are correct.
    c. Only 2 and 4 are correct.
    d. Only 4 is correct.
    e. All are correct.

96. Linear attenuation coefficient will have the greatest effect on which CT image property?

    1. CT number
    2. noise
    3. contrast
    4. spatial resolution

    a. Only 1, 2, and 3 are correct.
    b. Only 1 and 3 are correct.
    c. Only 2 and 4 are correct.
    d. Only 4 is correct.
    e. All are correct.

97. Selection of reconstruction filter will have an effect on which CT property?

    1. noise
    2. spatial resolution
    3. contrast resolution
    4. CT number

    a. Only 1, 2, and 3 are correct.
    b. Only 1 and 3 are correct.
    c. Only 2 and 4 are correct.
    d. Only 4 is correct.
    e. All are correct.

98. The choice of pixel size in CT represents a compromise between noise and

    a. energy resolution.
    b. spatial resolution.
    c. contrast resolution.
    d. slice thickness.
    e. quantum mottle.

99. The Hounsfield unit (HU) for water is zero. The Hounsfield unit (HU) for bone and air are ____ and ____ respectively.

    a. $+500$ and -500
    b. -200 and $+100$
    c. $+700$ and -700
    d. -1000 and $+1000$
    e. $+1000$ and -1000

100. In CT imagers, x-rays interact primarily by the Compton effect. If the density of fat is 0.92 gm/cm^3 and the density of muscle is 1.04 cm/cm^3, the respective Hounsfield unit (HU) values are approximately

    a. $+100$ and $+200$.
    b. $+80$ and $+40$.
    c. $+40$ and -40.
    d. -40 and $+40$.
    e. -80 and $+40$.

101. After injection of contrast medium, the CT number for a region of the brain changes from 10 HU to 20 HU. This represents what increase in the linear attenuation coefficient?

    a. 1%.
    b. 5%.
    c. 10%.
    d. 20%.
    e. 100%.

102. A pelvis is imaged with CT. The CT numbers between the iliac bones are significantly decreased. The most reasonable explanation for this observation is

    a. high fat content.
    b. aliasing.
    c. detector failure.
    d. beam hardening.
    e. volume averaging.

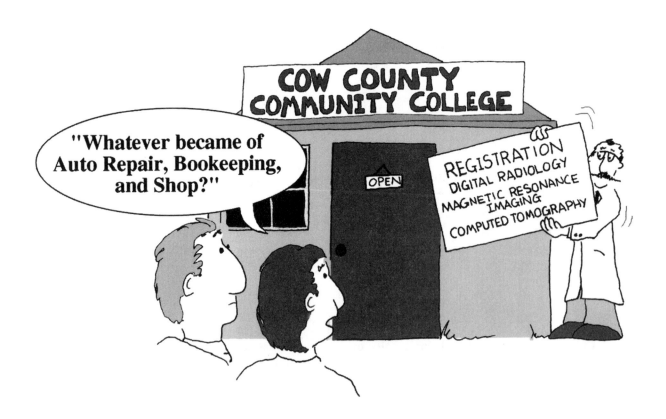

Spiral CT

- Continuous source rotation with patient translation through x-ray beam.

- Patient couch moves as x-ray tube rotates.

- High voltage supplied by **slip rings** or on-board generator.

- Slip rings replace cables.

- No interscan delay.

- Volumetric imaging within one breathhold, at least 25 s.

- Hyperventilation may help patients extend breathhold.

- Contrast-enhanced examination requires less contrast media.

- Detector data transferred to computer by slip rings.

- Examination time is greatly reduced.

- Patient comfort is much improved.

- Because the patient is moved through the gantry while the x-ray tube rotates, a spiral pattern results.

computed tomography
- source moves, detectors maybe
- source energized for 360°
- source stops, starts,...
- patient moves in

Spiral CT:
- source moves, detectors maybe, patient
- movement is continuous for entire examination

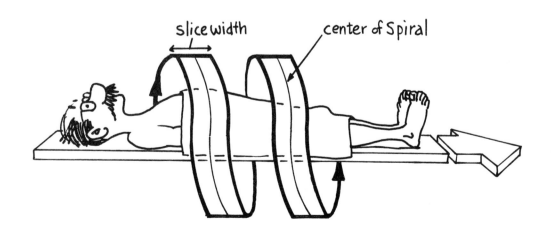

slice width   center of Spiral

$$\text{Spiral CT pitch} = \frac{\text{patient translation}/360°}{\text{slice thickness}}$$

Extended Spiral
Pitch = 2

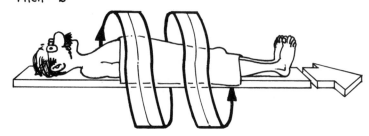

Contiguous Spiral
Pitch = 1

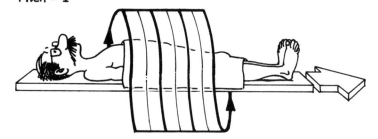

Overlapping Spiral
Pitch = 0.5

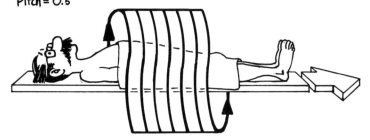

pitch	dose
0.5	X 2
1	X 1
1.5	X 0.7
2.0	X 0.5

- Z-axis resolution is slightly reduced with spiral CT.

- Effective slice thickness increases with pitch.

PITCH

- Pitch is the patient couch movement per rotation divided by slice thickness.

- Contiguous spiral: pitch = 1, that is, 10 mm/10 mm.

- Extended spiral: pitch = 2, that is, 20 mm/10 mm.

- Overlapping spiral: pitch = 1/2, that is, 5 mm/10 mm.

- Low pitch results in better z-axis resolution.

- Narrow collimation/low pitch results in better z-axis resolution than wide collimation/low pitch.

- Narrow collimation/low pitch is recommended for high contrast, thin slice examination, for example, lung nodules.

- Data is collected continuously but not from a transverse plane.

- As spiral CT pitch increases, patient dose is reduced.

- Patient dose is approximately proportional to 1/pitch.

- Patient dose is proportional to slice thickness divided by couch movement.

- Pitch in excess of 2 is not recommended for any clinical examination.

- Couch incrementation is usually set to equal collimation ∴ pitch = 1.

- Couch speed (mm/s) should not exceed slice thickness (mm) in order to obtain best compromise between image quality and image volume.

- Couch speed will not normally exceed 10 mm/s.

- When pitch exceeds 1, 180 interpolation must be used to limit loss of z-axis resolution.

- Longitudinal (z-axis) image coverage is the product of couch velocity (mm/s) and image time (s).

- The larger the pitch, the more anatomy is covered per examination.

INTERPOLATION

- Reconstruction of spiral CT images is the same as that for conventional CT except for interpolation.

- A transverse planar image can be reconstructed at any position along the axis of the patient (z-axis).

Spiral CT

pitch	couch move	slice thickness
½	1 mm	2 mm
½	2 mm	4 mm
½	5 mm	10 mm
1	5 mm	5 mm
1	10 mm	10 mm
2	4 mm	2 mm
2	10 mm	5 mm
2	20 mm	10 mm

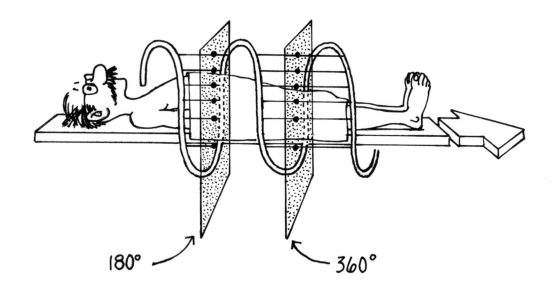

180°   360°

- The transverse image is reconstructed from spiral data first by interpolation, then by filtered back projection.

- Either 360° or 180° interpolation may be employed.

- Usually 180° interpolation is preferred.

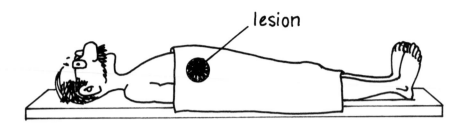

lesion

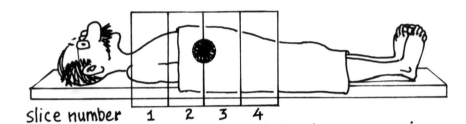

slice number 1 2 3 4
Conventional CT = partial volume averaging

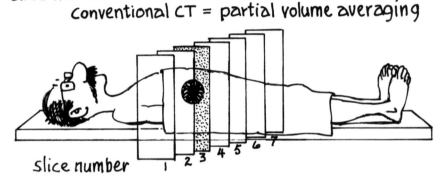

slice number 1 2 3 4 5 6 7

Spiral CT — overlapping reconstruction =
no partial volume averaging

Typical Collimation
  2-3 mm for CTA and lung nodules
  5 mm head and neck
  7-10 mm chest
  5-8 mm abdomen

- Contiguous reconstruction can result in partial volume effect when object is contained in adjacent slices.

- Overlapping reconstruction may be necessary to ensure that object is fully contained within a slice.

- Data acquisition is continuous along the z-axis; therefore by interpolation, image reconstruction is at any z-axis position.

- Regardless of z-axis position, slice thickness is determined by collimation.

- Volume averaging increases with increasing pitch.

- Image noise varies with spiral CT versus conventional CT depending on pitch.

- Interpolation is the computation of an unknown value using known values on either side.

- Z-axis resolution is improved with 180° interpolation compared to 360° interpolation.

- Extrapolation is the computation of an unknown value using known values on one side.

- 180° interpolation results in a thinner slice than 360° interpolation.

- 180° interpolation results in a noisier image than 360° interpolation.

- 180° interpolation results in approximately 20% higher noise than conventional CT.

- 360° interpolation results in approximately 20% less noise than conventional CT.

- 180° interpolation results in better z-axis resolution on reformatted longitudinal images than 360° interpolation.

- 180° interpolation allows scanning at a higher pitch than 360°.

- 360° interpolation broadens sensitivity profile more than 180° interpolation.

- In general, image noise is less for 360° interpolation, spiral CT than for conventional CT.

- In general, image noise is much higher for 180° interpolation, spiral CT than for conventional CT.

- Whether 180° or 360° interpolation, there are linear and higher order reconstruction algorithms.

- Two characteristic spiral CT artifacts have been identified as **breakup** and **stair step**.

- Both the breakup artifact and the stair step artifact occur as a consequence of reformatting interpolated transverse images to the longitudinal plane—coronal or sagittal.

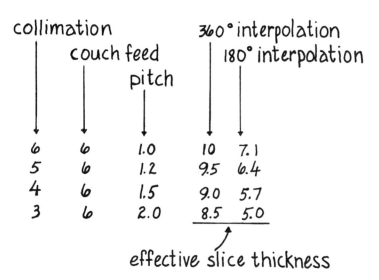

Approximate image noise

Conventional CT	100%
180° interpolation	125%
360° interpolation	85%

collimation	couch feed	pitch	360° interpolation	180° interpolation
6	6	1.0	10	7.1
5	6	1.2	9.5	6.4
4	6	1.5	9.0	5.7
3	6	2.0	8.5	5.0

effective slice thickness

pitch	effective slice thickness
½	no change
1	+ 10%
2	+ 30%
3	+ 70%

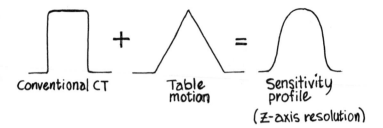

Conventional CT + Table motion = Sensitivity profile (z-axis resolution)

SENSITIVITY PROFILE

- Generally, when covering a given length of anatomy, thinner collimation and higher pitch are preferred because the result is better spatial resolution.

- Pitch greater than 2:1 is not clinically useful because of a broadened sensitivity profile and reduced z-axis resolution.

- Generally, higher pitch results in thinner slice thickness and less partial volume artifact.

- During spiral CT with pitch >1, the sensitivity profile (z-axis resolution) is wider than that of conventional CT.

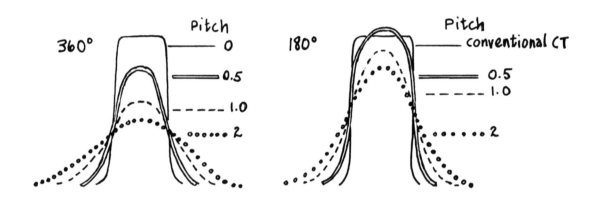

- Spiral CT sensitivity is described by the full width at tenth maximum (FWTM) rather than the conventional full width at half maximum (FWHM).

- The higher the pitch, the wider will be the sensitivity profile.

DESIGN FEATURES

SLIP RING TECHNOLOGY

- Slip ring technology made spiral CT possible.

- Normal spiral CT gantry rotation is 1 revolution per second.

- Although 0.5s revolution is possible, the engineering required by the stress of centrifugal force is formidable.

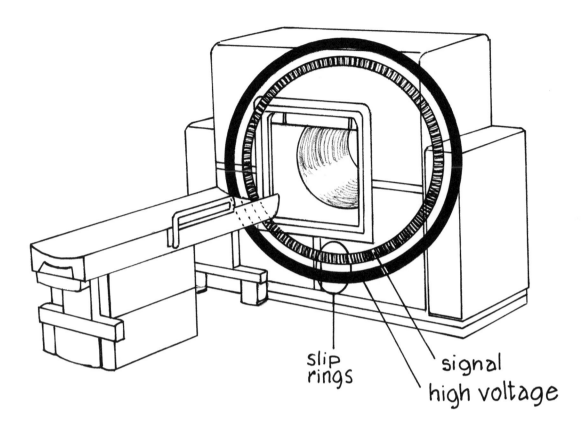

slip rings

signal
high voltage

- There may be multiple slip rings, both high voltage and low voltage.

- The design of spiral CT imagers is based on both third and fourth generation with no clear advantage to either.

- The slip ring contacts or brushes wear and are designed to be replaced during preventive maintenance.

X-RAY TUBE

- Spiral CT requires less than 1 s 360° rotation time and at least 5 MHU x-ray tubes.

- For very long scan times, mA must be reduced so that x-ray tube loading will not be exceeded.

- Regardless of heat capacity (MHU) and anode cooling (kHU/min), spiral CT is usually limited by the heat capacity of the focal track.

- High anode heat capacity (6-8 MHU) and rapid cooling (1 MHU/min) are required.

- In spite of the high heat load, tube life is comparable to conventional CT at about 50,000 exposures.

collimation	reconstruction	index
10 mm	10 mm	1.0
10 mm	5 mm	0.5
10 mm	1.5 mm	0.15

TECHNIQUE SELECTION

RECONSTRUCTION

- **Index** is the interval at which images are reconstructed.

- Index is reconstruction distance divided by collimation.

- An index of less than one indicates image overlap.

- An index of greater than one indicates a gap.

- An index of less than one should be employed to visualize suspected lung nodules.

- Spiral CT significantly improves coronal and sagittal slice reconstruction.

- High quality two-dimensional and three-dimensional image reformations are made from overlapping transverse images.

- Spiral CT operation requires the following unique technique selections: scan time, beam collimation, couch feed velocity, and z-axis spacing for image reconstruction.

- Spiral images cannot be reconstructed as rapidly as they are acquired. Hence, computer memory must be excessive.

- Scan time cannot exceed the patient's breath-hold capacity, usually about 25 s.

- Collimation and couch velocity can be selected as pitch.

Z-AXIS RESOLUTION

- Z-axis resolution is compromised in spiral CT but not significantly.

- The ability to reconstruct images at any z-axis location improves small lesion detection by reducing partial volume effects.

ADVANTAGES AND LIMITATIONS

- Image noise is usually less with spiral CT.

- More data is acquired in spiral CT; therefore, image reconstruction takes a little longer.

- Spiral CT replaces single scan techniques with volume acquisition techniques.

- Spiral CT misses no anatomy in the scanned volume.

- Spiral CT images can be reconstructed at any z-axis position.

- Multiple overlapping transverse images are possible in a single breathhold with no additional patient dose.

- Overall scan time is less with spiral CT resulting in improved patient throughput.

- Spiral CT takes a bit longer for image processing because of the required interpolation before planar image reconstruction.

Advantages:
Spiral CT v. Conventional CT
- faster image acquisition
- contrast can be followed quicker
- reduced patient dose at pitch > 1
- physiologic imaging
- improved 3D imaging
- angiographic imaging
- fewer partial volume artifacts
- freeze breathing
- fewer motion artifacts
- no misregistration
- increased throughput
- improved patient comfort
- variable reconstruction position
- real time CT biopsy

Chapter 5 Practice Questions

1. **A principal characteristic of spiral CT is**
   a. continuous rotation of the x-ray beam.
   b. high kVp.
   c. high mAs.
   d. multislice imaging.
   e. thin slice imaging.

2. **Which of the following has the poorest z-axis resolution?**
   a. conventional CT, 1 mm slice
   b. conventional CT, 5 mm slice
   c. spiral CT, 3 mm slice, pitch 0.5
   d. spiral CT, 3 mm slice, pitch 1
   e. spiral CT, 3 mm slice, pitch 2.0

3. **For spiral CT, the high-voltage cable an/or signal cable are replaced by**
   a. data acquisition system (DAS).
   b. high-frequency convolution algorithm.
   c. low-frequency convolution algorithm.
   d. no intrascan delay.
   e. slip rings.

4. One of the principal advantages of spiral CT over conventional CT is

   a. improved contrast resolution.
   b. improved image reconstruction.
   c. improved spatial resolution.
   d. no intrascan delay.
   e. volumetric imaging within one breathhold.

5. One procedure that can help patients extend their breathholding capacity is

   a. continuous patient translation.
   b. continuous x-ray tube rotation.
   c. hyperventilation.
   d. no intrascan delay.
   e. slip ring technology.

6. If one wishes to view images that are not contiguous

   a. a pitch of less than 1 is required.
   b. an index greater than 1 is required.
   c. couch movement in excess of 10 mm per second is required.
   d. gantry rotation of greater than 1 revolution per second is required.
   e. high-pass convolution filters should be employed.

7. One advantage of spiral CT over conventional CT is

   a. contrast resolution is improved.
   b. patients are more comfortable.
   c. spatial resolution is improved.
   d. the examination time is less.
   e. there is no intrascan delay.

8. The effective spiral pattern of the image results from

   a. continuous source rotation and patient translation.
   b. continuous source rotation and stepped patient translation.
   c. interpolation.
   d. no intrascan delay.
   e. reduced examination time.

9. When compared to conventional CT, which of the following applies to spiral CT?

   1. large volume data acquisition
   2. image reconstruction at any z-axis position with additional patient dose
   3. image reconstruction at any z-axis position with no additional patient dose
   4. skip scan technique

   a. Only 1, 2, and 3 are correct.
   b. Only 1 and 3 are correct.
   c. Only 2 and 4 are correct.
   d. Only 4 is correct.
   e. All are correct.

10. Which of the following is increased with increasing spiral CT pitch?

   a. axial resolution
   b. contrast resolution
   c. effective slice thickness
   d. image artifacts
   e. spatial resolution

11. With 10 mm slice collimation and a reconstruction interval of 5 mm, the spiral CT index is

    a. 0.5.
    b. 1.5.
    c. 2.
    d. 5.
    e. 10.

12. Which of the following is improved by spiral CT compared to conventional CT?

    1. more imaging volume
    2. less contrast medium
    3. shorter examination time
    4. patient comfort

    a. Only 1, 2, and 3 are correct.
    b. Only 1 and 3 are correct.
    c. Only 2 and 4 are correct.
    d. Only 4 is correct.
    e. All are correct.

13. Normal spiral CT gantry rotation is

    a. one revolution per second.
    b. one revolution per minute.
    c. two revolution per second.
    d. five revolutions per minute.
    e. ten revolutions per minute.

14. When a spiral CT exam is described as having a pitch of 1

    a. slice thickness is 10 mm divided by patient couch movement per revolution of 10 mm.
    b. slice thickness is 10 mm divided by patient couch movement per revolution of 5 mm.
    c. the patient couch will move 10 mm and slice thickness is 10 mm.
    d. the patient couch will move 10 mm and slice thickness is 5 mm per revolution.
    e. the patient couch will move 10 mm per revolution and slice thickness is 5 mm.

15. The principal reason spiral CT x-ray tubes require increased anode cooling (kHU per minute) is the

    a. efficient x-ray production.
    b. higher kVp employed.
    c. higher mA employed.
    d. long scan time.
    e. slip ring technology.

16. An overlapping spiral is one in which the

    a. pitch is 2.
    b. pitch is 1.
    c. pitch is 0.5.
    d. slice thickness is less than 10 mm.
    e. slice thickness is less than 20 mm.

17. A spiral CT exam is described as having a pitch of 2.

    a. The patient couch moves 20 mm per revolution and the slice thickness is 20 mm.
    b. The patient couch moves 20 mm per revolution and the slice thickness is 10 mm.
    c. The patient couch moves 20 mm per revolution and the slice thickness is 5 mm.
    d. Two revolutions are completed per each 10 mm couch increment.
    e. Two revolutions are completed per each 20 mm couch increment.

18. Index as applied to spiral CT is defined as

    a. couch movement per revolution.
    b. the degree employed for interpolation.
    c. the pitch divided by slice thickness.
    d. the range of extrapolation.
    e. the reconstruction distance divided by collimation.

19. Which of the following would be considered a contiguous spiral?

    1. couch movement per revolution 10 mm, slice thickness 10 mm
    2. couch movement per revolution 20 mm, slice thickness 10 mm
    3. couch movement per revolution 20 mm, slice thickness 20 mm
    4. couch movement per revolution 10 mm, slice thickness 20 mm

    a. Only 1, 2, and 3 are correct.
    b. Only 1 and 3 are correct.
    c. Only 2 and 4 are correct.
    d. Only 4 is correct.
    e. All are correct.

20. When comparing 180° interpolation with 360° interpolation,

    a. contrast resolution is better.
    b. image noise is less.
    c. reconstruction time is reduced.
    d. spatial resolution is better.
    e. thinner slices are possible.

21. The principal disadvantage of 180° extrapolation compared to 360° extrapolation is

    a. reduced z-axis resolution.
    b. reduced spatial resolution.
    c. reduced contrast resolution.
    d. more image noise.
    e. more image artifacts.

22. When high resolution imaging is desired, one should use

    a. high pitch with thin slice.
    b. high pitch with thick slice.
    c. low pitch with thin slice.
    d. low pitch with thick slice.
    e. variable pitch with variable slice.

23. A higher pitch in spiral CT results in
    a. better z-axis resolution.
    b. better spatial resolution.
    c. better contrast resolution.
    d. higher image noise.
    e. fewer artifacts.

24. Compared to conventional CT, spiral CT imaging with a pitch of 2 results in an effective slice thickness that is approximately
    a. 30% less.
    b. 10% less.
    c. the same
    d. 10% more.
    e. 30% more.

25. Which of the following is true for spiral CT compared to conventional CT?
    1. the source moves continuously
    2. spatial resolution is improved
    3. the patient moves continuously
    4. contrast resolution is improved

    a. Only 1, 2, and 3 are correct.
    b. Only 1 and 3 are correct.
    c. Only 2 and 4 are correct.
    d. Only 4 is correct.
    e. All are correct.

26. The recommended collimation for imaging lung nodules is approximately
    a. 1 mm.
    b. 2–3 mm
    c. 4–5 mm.
    d. 6–7 mm.
    e. 8–10 mm.

27. In spiral CT,
    1. data acquisition is continuous.
    2. data is acquired from a transverse plane.
    3. interpolation of data is required.
    4. z-axis resolution is improved.

    a. Only 1, 2, and 3 are correct.
    b. Only 1 and 3 are correct.
    c. Only 2 and 4 are correct.
    d. Only 4 is correct.
    e. All are correct.

28. Which of the following is likely to have the lowest patient dose? A pitch of
    a. 0.5.
    b. 1.
    c. 1.5.
    d. 2.
    e. 2.5.

29. The recommended collimation for imaging the head and neck is approximately

    a. 1 mm.

    b. 2–3 mm.

    c. 4–5 mm.

    d. 6–7 mm.

    e. 8–10.

30. Patient dose is approximately proportional to

    a. couch incrementation divided by rotation time.

    b. couch incrementation divided slice thickness.

    c. slice thickness divided by couch incrementation.

    d. slice thickness divided by pitch.

    e. slice thickness multiplied by couch incrementation.

31. What is the maximum spiral CT pitch recommended for a normal examination of the trunk?

    a. 0.5

    b. 1

    c. 1.5

    d. 2.

    e. 2.5

32. The maximum recommended couch speed during spiral CT is

    a. 5 mm per second.

    b. 10 mm per second.

    c. 15 mm per second.

    d. 20 mm per second.

    e. 30 mm per second.

33. Recommended collimation for computed tomography angiography (CTA) is approximately

    a. 1 mm.

    b. 2–3 mm

    c. 4–5 mm.

    d. 6–7 mm.

    e. 8–10 mm.

34. Longitudinal image coverage during spiral CT is the

    a. couch movement divided by image time.

    b. couch movement multiplied by pitch.

    c. image time divided by couch movement.

    d. image time multiplied by pitch.

    e. product of couch movement and image time.

35. If one wishes to image more anatomy, the principal technique change is

    a. increase collimation.

    b. increase pitch.

    c. increase scan time.

    d. reduce collimation.

    e. reduce pitch.

36. A spiral CT image differs from a step-and--shoot CT image because of
    a. back projected reconstruction.
    b. convolution filtering.
    c. interpolation.
    d. noise reduction.
    e. postprocessing.

37. Following a spiral CT examination and during postprocessing,
    a. patient translation can be selected.
    b. pitch can be selected.
    c. slice thickness can be selected.
    d. spatial resolution can be improved.
    e. any z-axis image position is possible.

38. The principal advantage that 180° interpolation has over 360° interpolation is
    a. better contrast resolution.
    b. better spatial resolution.
    c. better z-axis resolution.
    d. fewer image artifacts.
    e. less image noise.

39. If one wishes to reduce partial volume averaging during spiral CT, one should
    a. increase pitch.
    b. increase slice thickness.
    c. increase the patient dose.
    d. reduce pitch.
    e. reduce scan time.

40. Which of the following would be considered an overlapping spiral?
    1. couch movement per revolution 10 mm, slice thickness 10 mm
    2. couch movement per revolution 20 mm, slice thickness 20 mm
    3. couch movement per revolution 20 mm, slice thickness 10 mm
    4. couch movement per revolution 10 mm, slice thickness 20 mm

    a. Only 1, 2, and 3 are correct.
    b. Only 1 and 3 are correct.
    c. Only 2 and 4 are correct.
    d. Only 4 is correct.
    e. All are correct.

41. Which of the following best describes interpolation?
    a. averaging three or more known values
    b. estimating a value between two known values
    c. extending the range of vales to lower end
    d. extending the range of values to higher end
    e. transforming a set of values with a common coefficient

42. Which is the reconstruction algorithm usually preferred for spiral CT?
    a. 90° interpolation
    b. 180° interpolation
    c. 270° interpolation
    d. 360° interpolation
    e. incremental interpolation

43. When compared to conventional CT, spiral CT has
    a. better z-axis resolution.
    b. fewer artifacts.
    c. improved contrast resolution.
    d. improved spatial resolution.
    e. improved temporal resolution.

44. The recommended collimation for imaging the abdomen is approximately
    a. 1 mm.
    b. 2–3 mm.
    c. 4–5 mm.
    d. 6–7 mm.
    e. 8–10 mm.

45. Compared to conventional CT, spiral CT imaging with a pitch of 1 has an effective slice thickness that is approximately
    a. 30% less.
    b. 10% less.
    c. the same.
    d. 10% more.
    e. 30% more.

46. When comparing narrow collimation, low pitch to wide collimation, high pitch, the former has better
    1. spatial resolution.
    2. contrast resolution.
    3. z-axis resolution.
    4. image noise.

    a. Only 1, 2, and 3 are correct.
    b. Only 1 and 3 are correct.
    c. Only 2 and 4 are correct.
    d. Only 4 is correct.
    e. All are correct.

47. The most often employed spiral CT technique is
    a. couch incrementation each revolution.
    b. very narrow collimation.
    c. couch movement of 20 mm per second.
    d. use of pitch equal to 1.
    e. use of pitch equal to 2.

48. **Which technique is recommended for imaging calcified lung nodules?**

    a. incremental collimation, contiguous pitch
    b. narrow collimation, high pitch
    c. narrow collimation, low pitch
    d. wide collimation, high pitch
    e. wide collimation, low pitch

49. **In general terms, patient dose is**

    a. independent of pitch.
    b. independent of mA.
    c. independent of kVp.
    d. higher with increasing pitch.
    e. lower with increasing pitch.

50. **The recommended collimation for imaging the chest is approximately**

    a. 1 mm.
    b. 2–3 mm.
    c. 4–5 mm.
    d. 6–7 mm.
    e. 8–10 mm.

51. **Compared to conventional CT, spiral CT with a pitch of 0.5 results in a slice thickness that is approximately**

    a. 30% less.
    b. 10% less.
    c. the same.
    d. 10% more.
    e. 30% more.

52. **Which of the following would be considered an extended spiral?**

    1. couch movement per revolution 10 mm, slice thickness 5 mm
    2. couch movement per revolution 20 mm, slice thickness 10 mm
    3. couch movement per revolution 10 mm, slice thickness 8 mm
    4. couch movement per revolution 20 mm, slice thickness 14 mm

    a. Only 1, 2, and 3 are correct.
    b. Only 1 and 3 are correct.
    c. Only 2 and 4 are correct.
    d. Only 4 is correct.
    e. All are correct.

53. **When comparing 180° interpolation with 360° interpolation,**

    1. z-axis resolution is better.
    2. thinner slices are possible.
    3. image noise is increased.
    4. higher pitch scanning is possible.

    a. Only 1, 2, and 3 are correct.
    b. Only 1 and 3 are correct.
    c. Only 2 and 4 are correct.
    d. Only 4 is correct.
    e. All are correct.

54. **The lower the spiral CT pitch,**

    a. the fewer the resultant artifacts.
    b. the better the contrast resolution.
    c. the better the spatial resolution.
    d. the better the z-axis resolution.
    e. the lower the image noise.

55. **When compared to conventional CT,**

    a. spiral CT pitch greater than 1 results in a wider sensitivity profile.
    b. spiral CT pitch of 1 results in a wider sensitivity profile.
    c. spiral CT pitch of 0.5 results in a wider sensitivity profile.
    d. sensitivity profile is inversely proportional to pitch.
    e. sensitivity profile increases with decreasing pitch.

56. **The preferred description of spiral CT sensitivity profile is**

    a. full width at tenth maximum (FWTM).
    b. full width at half maximum (FWHM).
    c. full width at 0.7 maximum.
    d. prepatient collimation width.
    e. postpatient collimation width.

57. **Which of the following is improved by spiral CT compared to conventional CT?**

    1. axial resolution
    2. examination time
    3. spatial resolution
    4. larger imaging volume

    a. Only 1, 2, and 3 are correct.
    b. Only 1 and 3 are correct.
    c. Only 2 and 4 are correct.
    d. Only 4 is correct.
    e. All are correct.

58. **The anode heat capacity of a spiral CT x-ray tube is high principally because of the**

    a. efficient x-ray production.
    b. higher kVp employed.
    c. higher mA employed.
    d. long scan time.
    e. slip ring technology.

59. **An extended spiral is defined as one in which the**

    a. pitch is 2.
    b. pitch is 1.
    c. pitch is 0.5.
    d. slice thickness is greater than 10 mm.
    e. slice thickness is greater than 20 mm.

60. **The term "index" when applied to spiral CT is**

    a. couch movement per revolution.
    b. the degree employed for interpolation.
    c. the interval at which images are reconstructed.
    d. the pitch divided by slice thickness.
    e. the range of extrapolation.

61. **An overlapping spiral is one in which**

    a. the couch moves less than 10 mm per revolution.
    b. the couch moves less than 20 mm per revolution.
    c. the pitch is 0.5.
    d. the pitch is 1.0.
    e. the pitch is 2.0.

62. **If one wishes to view overlapping images,**

    a. a pitch of less than 1 is required.
    b. an index of less than 1 is required.
    c. couch movement in excess of 10 mm per second is required.
    d. gantry rotation of greater than 1 revolution per second is required.
    e. high-pass convolution filters should be employed.

63. **When compared to conventional CT, spiral CT**

    a. has improved contrast resolution.
    b. has improved spatial resolution.
    c. has less noise.
    d. produces fewer artifacts.
    e. requires less contrast media.

64. **Which of the following represents significant image improvement with spiral CT compared to conventional CT?**

    1. better coronal and sagittal image reconstruction
    2. improved z-axis resolution
    3. larger tissue volume imaged
    4. shorter x-ray beam-on time

    a. Only 1, 2, and 3 are correct.
    b. Only 1 and 3 are correct.
    c. Only 2 and 4 are correct.
    d. Only 4 is correct.
    e. All are correct.

65. **Spiral CT pitch is defined as**

    a. field of view (FOV) divided by slice thickness.
    b. patient translation divided by field of view (FOV).
    c. patient translation divided by slice thickness.
    d. patient translation multiplied by field of view (FOV).
    e. patient translation multiplied by slice thickness.

66. With a slice collimation of 5 mm and a reconstruction distance of 10 mm, the spiral CT index is

   a. 0.5.
   b. 1.5.
   c. 2.
   d. 5.
   e. 10.

67. Spiral CT of the thorax should not exceed the breathhold capacity of the patient. Normally, this is approximately

   a. 5 seconds.
   b. 10 seconds.
   c. 15 seconds.
   d. 25 seconds.
   e. 50 seconds.

68. Which of the following is somewhat reduced with spiral CT compared to conventional CT?

   a. axial resolution
   b. contrast resolution
   c. effective slice thickness
   d. image noise
   e. spatial resolution

69. A principal characteristic of spiral CT is

   a. high kVp.
   b. high mAs.
   c. multislice imaging.
   d. patient translation through the x-ray beam
   e. thin slice imaging.

70. When compared to conventional CT, which of the following applies to spiral CT?

   1. better z-axis resolution
   2. less partial volume effect
   3. less image noise
   4. longer image reconstruction time

   a. Only 1, 2, and 3 are correct.
   b. Only 1 and 3 are correct.
   c. Only 2 and 4 are correct.
   d. Only 4 is correct.
   e. All are correct.

71. When one selects a particular spiral CT pitch, the selection involves

   a. collimation and couch movement.
   b. collimation and index.
   c. couch movement and field of view.
   d. index and interpolation algorithm.
   e. interpolation algorithm and couch movement.

72. **When compared to conventional CT, which of the following applies to spiral CT?**
    1. longer image processing
    2. skip scan technique
    3. shorter patient throughput
    4. higher image noise

    a. Only 1, 2, and 3 are correct.
    b. Only 1 and 3 are correct.
    c. Only 2 and 4 are correct.
    d. Only 4 is correct.
    e. All are correct.

73 **One advantage of spiral CT is**
    1. that contrast media can be followed quicker.
    2. reduced patient dose at pitch less than 1.
    3. improved patient throughput.
    4. enhanced misregistration.

    a. Only 1, 2, and 3 are correct.
    b. Only 1 and 3 are correct.
    c. Only 2 and 4 are correct.
    d. Only 4 is correct.
    e. All are correct.

74. **The principal characteristics of spiral CT include**
    a. patient couch moves as the examination is in progress.
    b. multiple detector arrays are employed.
    c. multiple x-ray tubes are employed.
    d. postprocessing is eliminated.
    e. longitudinal resolution is approved.

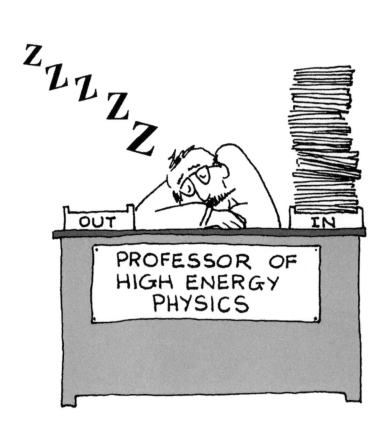

Special Imaging Techniques

DYNAMIC COMPUTED TOMOGRAPHY

- **Dynamic scanning** implies 15 or more scans in rapid sequence within one minute.

- Dynamic scanning is used for trauma, cardiac, and vascular imaging.

- Dynamic scanning allows imaging in the arterial phase following bolus injection.

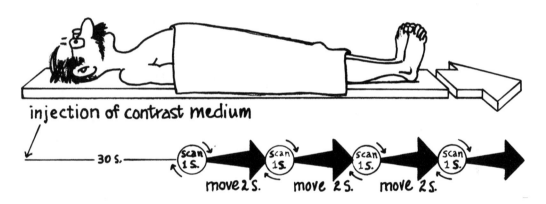

injection of contrast medium

30 s.   scan 1 s.   move 2 s.   scan 1 s.   move 2 s.   scan 1 s.   move 2 s.   scan 1 s.

- Typical dynamic scanning would be 15 one-second scans, each separated by a two-second interscan time during which the couch would increment a distance equal to the slice thickness.

- Tube cooling will limit the extent of dynamic scanning.

- Dynamic scanning has been largely replaced by spiral CT.

- Spiral CT permits imaging of the entire liver and pancreas at a specified time phase such as arterial, portal, or venous.

- **Computed tomography (CT) guided biopsy** is performed to localize using a region of interest (ROI) feature.

- Radiopaque markers are used to help guide needle to the area of interest.

Typical abdominal Spiral CT
- must complete examination within one breathhold
- 10 mm slice thickness
- 5 mm/s couch movement
- for liver-pancreas, start imaging 40s after 150 ml bolus at 3 ml/s

Typical chest spiral CT
- must complete examination within one breathhold
- 10 mm slice thickness
- 15-20 mm/s couch movement
- follow-up with thinner slice spiral CT of suspicious tissue

- Wide window width (WW = 500 to 1000), low window level (WL = 40 to 60) for bone imaging.

- Wide WW (= 700 to 900), high WL (= 800) for lung imaging.

- Narrow WW (= 200 to 400), low WL (= 40 to 60) for abdomen and pelvis imaging.

- Computed tomography fluoroscopy provides 8 images/second for near real-time imaging.

- Computed tomography fluoroscopy is most useful for angiointervention in the abdomen and chest.

- Computed tomography fluoroscopy results in high patient and personnel dose.

- Computed tomography fluoroscopy is particularly helpful for CT-guided biopsy.

- Patient dose during CT fluoroscopy is kept low by using low mA, 30 mA.

QUANTITATIVE COMPUTED TOMOGRAPHY (QCT)

- Quantitative computed tomography employs an ROI to determine the average CT number of a tissue as an aid to diagnosis.

- Quantitative computed tomography can be helpful in characterizing a tumor.

- Quantitative computed tomography can distinguish between cystic and solid lesions.

- With spirometric control and breath-triggered imaging, QCT can measure the density and characterize the structure of lung tissue.

- Quantitative CT is very helpful for measuring tissue perfusion following bolus injection of an iodinated contrast media.

- Quantitative computed tomography allows measurement of cerebral blood flow following xenon inhalation.

HEART SCAN

- Electron beam CT (EBCT) of the heart can reveal plaque volume and calcium content in coronary arteries.

- Electron beam CT of the heart is a cost-effective screening for coronary artery disease with no patient discomfort.

- A typical heart scan consists of 40 ECG-triggered 3 mm images acquired at 100 ms each.

- Calcium is a natural marker in athersclerotic plagues making EBCT an effective screening device.

COMPUTED TOMOGRAPHY ANGIOGRAPHY (CTA)

- Computed tomography angiography (CTA) allows maximum visualization of the pulmonary artery and its segmental branches.

- Stroke is the highest cause of morbidity and the third highest cause of mortality.

- Computed tomography angiography requires low kVp and mA, for example, 90 kVp/100mA.

- Computed tomography angiography is best performed with spiral CT.

- Unlike MRA, CTA is not susceptible to motion or flow artifacts.

- Computed tomography angiography is much less invasive and lower in dose than a conventional angiogram.

- Bone is removed from CTA maximum intensity projection (MIP) image by an editing procedure called **image segmentation**.

- Computed tomography angiography requires less film than conventional angiography.

- Computed tomography angiography requires less staff than conventional angiography.

- Computed tomography angiography requires less contrast media than conventional angiography.

- Computed tomography angiography is at least a factor of two less expensive than conventional angiography.

- Computed tomography angiography employs MIP and multiplanar reconstruction (MPR) to maximum advantage.

- Computed tomography angiography success depends on collimation, pitch, vessel orientation, and reconstruction interval.

Typical head and neck spiral CT
- less affected by respiratory motion
- 2.5 mm slice thickness
- 1.5 mm/s couch movement
- start imaging 50s following bolus injection
- 100 mL contrast media injected at 1-2 mL/s

advantages of CTA:
- non-invasive
- examination time in seconds
- can image patients with aneurysm clips
- analyze vessel wall and lumen
- multiplanar imaging
- central contrast media injection of 15cc or less
- can be performed as emergency
- less expensive than conventional angiography
- less dose than conventional angiography

disadvantages of CTA:
- depends on hardware/software
- may need a separate post-processing work station
- classic CT artifacts
- best spatial resolution 0.3mm (2 lp/cm)

MULTISLICE IMAGING (MI)

- This development was first produced by Elscint and is now available from all CT manufacturers.

- Multislice imaging incorporates two or more contiguous detector arrays.

- Multislice imaging produces two or more section images simultaneously.

- Multislice imaging is a spiral CT technique.

- Multislice imaging greatly reduces imaging time, from approximately 3 minutes with conventional CT to less than 30 seconds.

Four contiguous simultaneous slices

Four detector arrays

- The main advantage to MI is faster imaging with better spatial resolution.

- Complete x-ray tube/detector array rotation in less than 1 s.

- Partial scan images can be obtained in approximately 100 ms.

- Best imaging requires a pitch of 3:1 to 6:1.

- Multislice imaging requires exceptional engineering because of the mechanical forces produced by gantry rotation.

- Image reconstruction uses 360° interpolation rather than 180° interpolation.

- 360° interpolation of multislice images allows faster imaging with improved spatial and temporal resolution and reduced noise.

- Misregistration of anatomy is reduced because of the faster patient couch speed.

- Motion artifacts are greatly reduced.

- Patient breathhold is much less demanding.

- Imaging larger z-axis volume in less time is possible with MI.

- Less contrast medium is required.

- Patient throughput is increased with MI.

- Variable slice thickness can be produced with postprocessing. In many cases, rescan is unnecessary because of postprocessing.

- Computed tomography angiography is greatly improved with MI.

- Because of imaging speed, coronary artery calcification assay with MI is a challenge to EBCT.

Chapter 6 Practice Questions

1. **Dynamic scanning is a term applied to**
   a. 15 or more conventional CT scans in rapid succession.
   b. high pitch spiral CT scanning.
   c. lower pitch spiral CT scanning.
   d. overlapping scans.
   e. zero interscan.

2. **In CT imaging, the ability to see a small density difference between adjacent large objects, all other factors constant, is increased by**
   1. reducing the focal spot.
   2. reducing the scanning time.
   3. reducing the absorption efficiency of the detectors.
   4. increasing the dose.

   a. Only 1, 2, and 3 are correct.
   b. Only 1 and 3 are correct.
   c. Only 2 and 4 are correct.
   d. Only 4 is correct.
   e. All are correct.

3. **Dynamic scanning is particularly useful in which of the following?**
   1. trauma
   2. skeletal
   3. cardiac
   4. abdomen

   a. Only 1, 2, and 3 are correct.
   b. Only 1 and 3 are correct.
   c. Only 3 and 4 are correct.
   d. Only 4 is correct.
   e. All are correct.

4. Electron beam CT finds principal application in imaging
   a. abdomen.
   b. bone.
   c. brain.
   d. heart.
   e. lungs.

5. A principal advantage to CTA compared to MRA is
   a. three-dimensional reconstruction is not possible.
   b. imaging time is increased.
   c. no flow artifacts.
   d. postprocessing is limited.
   e. shaded surface reconstruction is not possible.

6. Which of the following are particularly aided by quantitative computed tomography (QCT)?
   1. determining cystic or solid
   2. assisting in needle biopsy
   3. measuring tissue perfusion
   4. imaging at reduced patient dose

   a. Only 1, 2, and 3 are correct.
   b. Only 1 and 3 are correct.
   c. Only 2 and 4 are correct.
   d. Only 4 is correct.
   e. All are correct.

7. Compared to conventional angiography, computed tomography angiography (CTA)
   1. has better spatial resolution.
   2. has better contrast resolution.
   3. requires higher patient dose.
   4. is less expensive.

   a. Only 1, 2, and 3 are correct.
   b. Only 1 and 3 are correct.
   c. Only 2 and 4 are correct.
   d. Only 4 is correct.
   e. All are correct.

8. QCT stands for
   a. quantitative computed tomography.
   b. quality computed tomography.
   c. quantity computed tomography.
   d. question computed tomography.
   e. quick computed tomography.

9. **A characteristic of electron beam CT (EBCT) is**

    1. 100 ms imaging.
    2. imaging with electrons.
    3. reduced motion blur.
    4. improved spatial resolution.

    a. Only 1, 2, and 3 are correct.
    b. Only 1 and 3 are correct.
    c. Only 2 and 4 are correct.
    d. Only 4 is correct.
    e. All are correct.

10. **Successful quantitative computed tomography (QCT)**

    a. depends on at least two different kVp.
    b. is a method of reducing CT imaging time.
    c. is postprocessing to reduce image artifacts.
    d. requires a spiral CT imager.
    e. requires a region of interest (ROI).

11. **The principal limitations to dynamic CT imaging is**

    a. available postprocessing.
    b. maximum field of view (FOV).
    c. patient movement.
    d. scan aperture.
    e. x-ray tube cooling.

12. **Quantitative computed tomography (QCT) is principally employed to**

    a. determine tissue CT number
    b. establish a region of interest (ROI).
    c. estimate organ size.
    d. estimate organ volume.
    e. present image reversal.

13. **Compared to conventional angiography, computed tomography angiography (CTA)**

    1. allows three-dimensional reconstruction.
    2. has lower patient dose.
    3. is less invasive.
    4. has better spatial resolution.

    a. Only 1, 2, and 3 are correct.
    b. Only 1 and 3 are correct.
    c. Only 2 and 4 are correct.
    d. Only 4 is correct.
    e. All are correct.

14. **Dynamic scanning is employed when**

    a. fast imaging is required.
    b. high contrast resolution imaging is required.
    c. high spatial resolution imaging is required.
    d. patient motion is a problem.
    e. spiral CT is not available.

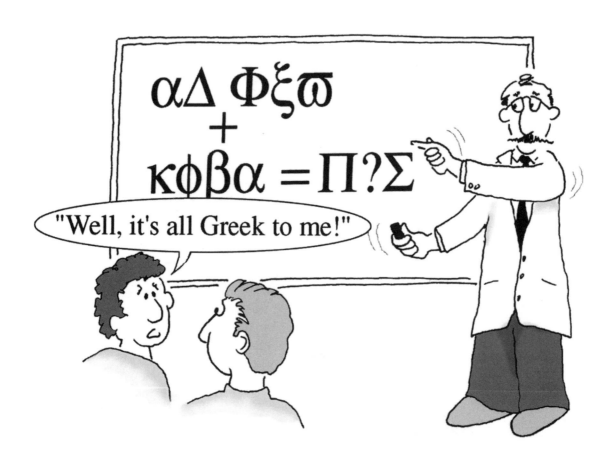

Image Quality

- Image quality can be described by five characteristics—contrast resolution, spatial resolution, image noise, linearity, and uniformity.

- Specification of image quality is usually very subjective and is described by terms such as detail, recorded detail, and sharpness or blur.

- Image quality cannot be represented correctly by a single number.

- Image quality can be represented by several numbers.

- Image quality can be described numerically by contrast resolution, spatial resolution, image noise, linearity, and uniformity.

CONTRAST RESOLUTION

- Contrast resolution describes the property of distinguishing between similar tissues, for example gray-white matter in brain and liver–spleen.

- Computed tomography (CT) imaging excels at contrast resolution.

- Contrast resolution with x-ray imaging is determined by tissue atomic number (Z), mass density $\rho(kg/m^3)$, and electron density (e/m^3).

- Tissues with a large difference in Z and ρ will have high contrast.

- During radiographic imaging, contrast resolution is improved with reduced scatter radiation and lower kVp.

- Computed tomography employs high kVp to minimize patient dose.

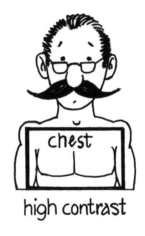

high contrast

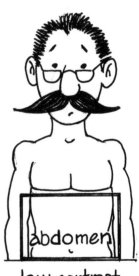

low contrast

contrast resolution is improved by:
- large pixel size
- high mAs
- thick slice
- low pass filter

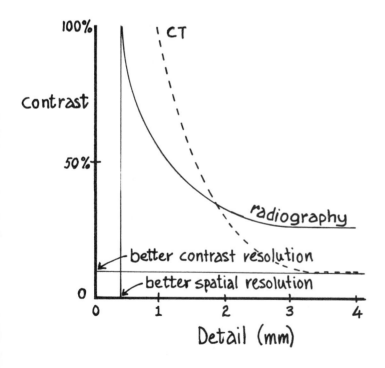

- Computed tomography imaging has superior contrast resolution because of narrow x-ray beam collimation, and therefore, excellent scatter radiation rejection.

- The larger the dynamic range, for example, 2^{10} (1024) versus 2^9 (512), the less contrast in the image.

- At low spatial frequencies the modulation transfer function (MTF) is a measure of contrast resolution.

- Contrast resolution is the ability to image adjacent tissues having a similar mass density and effective atomic number.

- Contrast resolution is improved by using higher mA.

- Contrast resolution is improved by imaging thicker slices.

- Contrast resolution is improved when imaging smaller patients.

- Contrast resolution is better with low noise imagers.

- Contrast resolution is improved with larger field of view (FOV) and smaller matrix size—hence, larger pixels.

- Contrast resolution can be improved with a smoothing reconstruction filter.

SPATIAL RESOLUTION

- Spatial resolution refers to the ability to faithfully reproduce small objects having high subject contrast.

- The bone–soft tissue interface represents very high subject contrast.

- The liver–spleen interface represents very low subject contrast.

- Spatial resolution is often described by the degree of blurring in an image.

- A bone–soft tissue interface will be very sharp and is described as a high spatial frequency interface.

- High spatial frequency objects are more difficult to image than low spatial frequency objects.

- Small, high contrast objects are more difficult to image than large, low contrast objects.

- Larger pixel size results in poorer spatial resolution.

- Lower subject contrast results in poorer spatial resolution.

- Larger detector size results in poorer spatial resolution.

- Larger prepatient and postpatient collimation results in more scatter radiation.

- Scatter radiation reduces contrast and results in less contrast resolution.

- A smaller x-ray tube focal spot improves spatial resolution because of the sharper image projection, not the geometry of a shadow.

- Point response function (PRF) is one method of evaluating spatial resolution.

- Edge response function (ERF) is one method of evaluating spatial resolution.

- Line spread function (LSF) is one method of evaluating spatial resolution.

- The Fourier transform (FT) is a mathematical manipulation to convert an intensity versus distance relationship into an intensity versus 1/distance (spatial frequency) relationship.

- The FT of a PRF results in the MTF.

- The FT of an ERF results in the MTF.

- The FT of a LSF results in the MTF.

- Spatial resolution is best described by the limiting spatial frequency (lp/cm).

- The MTF is obtained from the FT of the PSF, LSF, or the ERF.

- The MTF is useful when evaluating components of a system or comparing similar systems.

- Spatial resolution is improved with a smaller x-ray focal spot size.

spatial resolution is improved by:
- small detector size
- small pixel size
- thin slice
- high frequency convolution filter

low spatial frequency

1 lp

high spatial frequency

Q: what sized object can be resolved if the spatial resolution is 2 lp/mm ?

A: $\dfrac{2\ lp/mm = 4\ objects/mm}{(4\ objects/mm)} = 0.25\ mm$ object

point object
PRF
image

edge object
ERF
image

line object
LSF
image

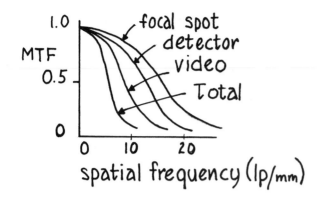

Object size	=	spatial frequency
0.1 mm		5 lp/mm
0.2 mm		2.5 lp/mm
0.5 mm		1.0 lp/mm
1.0 mm		0.5 lp/mm
2.0 mm		0.25 lp/mm
5.0 mm		0.1 lp/mm
10.0 mm		0.05 lp/mm

Mass Density of Various Tissue

Tissue	Mass Density (kg/m³)
Lung	320
Fat	910
Muscle	1000
Bone	1850

Effective Atomic Numbers of Various Tissue

Tissue	Effective Atomic Number
Fat	6.3
Muscle	7.4
Lung	7.4
Bone	13.8

- Spatial resolution is improved with thinner section imaging.

- Spatial resolution is improved with narrow predetector collimation.

- Spatial resolution is improved with longer source to isocenter distance.

- Spatial resolution can be improved with the use of an edge enhancement (convolution) reconstruction algorithm.

- Spatial resolution is improved by increasing the number of projection profiles acquired per scan.

- Spatial resolution is improved when smaller FOV or larger matrix size is employed.

- At high spatial frequencies the MTF is a measure of spatial resolution.

- The MTF is the principal means of expressing CT spatial resolution.

- To understand MTF, one must first understand spatial frequency, which has units of line pairs/mm (lp/mm).

- One line and a line-sized interspace is a one-line pair (lp).

- High spatial frequencies represent small objects.

- Low spatial frequencies represent large objects.

- An MTF value of 1.0 represents an absolutely perfect image.

- As MTF value is reduced, image blur increases and therefore image quality is reduced.

- Usually, the spatial frequency at the 0.1 (10%) MTF is identified as the limiting resolution.

- The total MTF of an imager is the product of component MTFs.

- Computed tomography imagers are capable of approximately 10 lp/cm (1 lp/mm) in normal mode and up to approximately 20 lp/cm (2 lp/mm) in the high resolution mode.

- Z-axis resolution is better with spiral CT compared to conventional CT.

IMAGE NOISE

- Contrast resolution is limited by image noise.

- Scatter radiation results in image noise.

- An increase in slice thickness results in less noise.

- An increase in slice thickness usually results in lower patient dose.

- An increase in pixel size results in less noise.

- An increase in patient dose results in less noise.

- In statistics, noise is called standard deviation and is symbolized by σ.

- High noise images appear blotchy, grainy, or spotty.

- Low noise images appear very smooth.

- Noise in a CT image comes from the scanner electronics and the random nature of x-ray interaction with a detector.

- Anything that will improve contrast resolution will reduce CT noise.

- Anything that reduces CT noise will improve contrast resolution.

- Increased image noise at low mAs can usually be accommodated by using a low-pass convolution filter.

- Image noise can be reduced by using 360° interpolation.

LINEARITY

- When water = 0, bone = 1000, and air = −1000, a CT imager exhibits perfect linearity.

- The CT number for a given tissue is determined by the x-ray linear attenuation coefficient (μ).

- A plot of CT number versus μ should be a straight line passing through water = 0.

- Good linearity is essential for **quantitative computed tomography (QCT)**.

- Linearity is the ability of the CT imager to assign the correct Hounsfield unit (HU) to a given tissue.

σ is a measure of noise

$$\sigma = \sqrt{\frac{\Sigma(\bar{x} - x_i)^2}{n-1}}$$

where x = CT number
n = number averaged

noise is reduced by increasing:
- mAs
- pixel size
- slice thickness

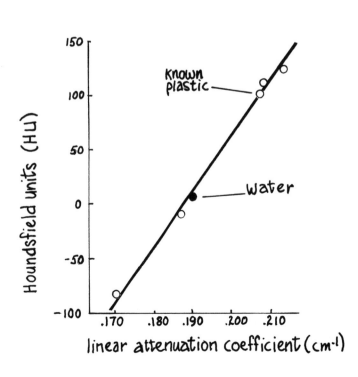

- Linearity is monitored by imaging the 5-pin insert of the American Association of Physicists in Medicine (AAPM) and plotting HU versus linear attenuation coefficient.

UNIFORMITY

- When a test object made of one substance is imaged, the value of each pixel should be the same.

- **Cupping** is the reduction in CT number toward the middle of a uniform test object.

- **Peaking** is the increase in CT number toward the middle of a uniform test object.

- Cupping and peaking are signs of poor image uniformity.

- Image uniformity is essential for QCT.

- Uniformity is the ability of the CT imager to assign the same HU to a uniform phantom (water) over the entire FOV.

CONTRAST-DETAIL

- Contrast-detail plots are instructive when evaluating contrast resolution and spatial resolution.

- Contrast-detail plots are useful when comparing different scanning protocols.

- The low contrast region of the contrast-detail curve is noise limited.

- The high contrast region of the contrast-detail curve is determined by the MTF of the imager components.

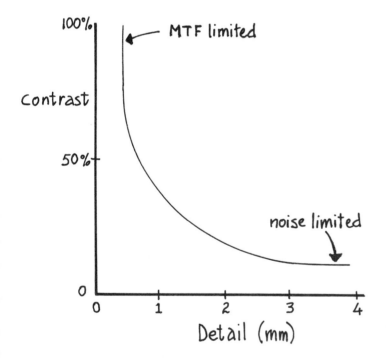

Chapter 7 Practice Questions

1. Which of the following are included in the principal characteristics of a medical image?

   1. spatial resolution
   2. contrast resolution
   3. image noise
   4. artifacts

   a. Only 1, 2, and 3 are correct.
   b. Only 1 and 3 are correct.
   c. Only 2 and 4 are correct.
   d. Only 4 is correct.
   e. All are correct.

2. Quantitative computed tomography (QCT) especially requires which of the following image characteristics?

   a. uniformity
   b. linearity
   c. spatial resolution
   d. contrast resolution
   e. low noise

3. Contrast resolution is improved most easily by

   a. increasing kVp.
   b. increasing mA.
   c. increasing (ROI) region of interest.
   d. reducing FOV (FOV).
   e. reducing slice thickness.

4. The term "peaking" in a CT image refers to

   a. an artifact induced by improper beam filtration.
   b. an artifact produced by improper (ROI) region of interest.
   c. the appropriate value of Hounsfield unit (HU) in multiple test objects.
   d. the constant value of Hounsfield unit (HU) in a uniform test object.
   e. the increase in CT number in the middle of a uniform test object.

5. Contrast resolution during projection radiography is compromised principally because of

   a. contrast media.
   b. imaging time.
   c. kVp.
   d. mA.
   e. scatter radiation.

6. "Peaking" artifact in a CT image is an example of

   a. poor contrast resolution.
   b. poor image linearity.
   c. poor image uniformity.
   d. poor spatial resolution.
   e. reconstruction algorithm mismatch.

7. **The principal reason to use high kVp during CT examination is**

    a. fewer artifacts.
    b. improved contrast resolution.
    c. improved spatial resolution.
    d. reduced image noise.
    e. reduced patient dose.

8. **Which of the following would be characteristic of a CT imager with perfect linearity?**

    1. a water value of 0
    2. a bone value of 1000
    3. an air value of -1000
    4. a straight line plot of CT number versus μ

    a. Only 1, 2, and 3 are correct.
    b. Only 1 and 3 are correct.
    c. Only 2 and 4 are correct.
    d. Only 4 is correct.
    e. All are correct.

9. **Which of the following is effective in improving contrast resolution in CT?**

    1. imaging thicker slices
    2. imaging bigger patients
    3. use a larger field of view (FOV)
    4. reduced pixel size

    a. Only 1, 2, and 3 are correct.
    b. Only 1 and 3 are correct.
    c. Only 2 and 4 are correct.
    d. Only 4 is correct.
    e. All are correct.

10. **Increasing the dynamic range of a CT image**

    a. improves image uniformity.
    b. improves spatial resolution.
    c. provides better image linearity.
    d. reduces image noise.
    e. results in more shades of gray.

11. **During CT examination, the principal x-ray interaction is**

    a. beam hardening.
    b. coherent scattering.
    c. Compton scattering.
    d. filtered back projection.
    e. photoelectric effect.

12. The value of the modulation transfer function (MTF) at low spatial frequencies is principally related to

    a. contrast resolution.
    b. image linearity.
    c. image noise.
    d. image uniformity.
    e. spatial resolution.

13. Image uniformity refers to

    a. accurate CT numbers.
    b. constant field of view (FOV).
    c. constant patient aperture.
    d. maximum intensity projection (MIP).
    e. one CT number value of a given object.

14. Spatial resolution in CT is approximately 1 lp/cm. What is the smallest sized object that can be imaged?

    a. 0.1 mm
    b. 0.25 mm
    c. 0.5 mm
    d. 1 mm
    e. 5 mm

15. One definition of contrast resolution is the

    a. ability to distinguish a small tissue from a larger one.
    b. ability to distinguish tissues having similar mass density.
    c. change in tissue appearance with kVp.
    d. rejection of scatter radiation.
    e. smallest object that can be imaged.

16. What feature of the CT image is principally limited by increasing image noise?

    a. artifacts
    b. contrast resolution
    c. imaging uniformity
    d. spatial resolution
    e. z-axis resolution

17. Which of the following has less image noise?

    a. 180° spiral CT
    b. 360° spiral CT
    c. conventional CT
    d. conventional CT reformatted
    e. z-axis reconstructed conventional CT

18. Contrast resolution can be improved by

    a. imaging smaller patients.
    b. using higher kVp.
    c. imaging faster.
    d. using a bone reconstruction filter.
    e. a reduced field of view.

19. **Computed tomography image noise can usually be reduced with**
    1. 360° interpolation rather than 180° interpolation.
    2. reduced scatter radiation.
    3. use of a low-frequency convolution filter.
    4. better image linearity.

    a. Only 1, 2, and 3 are correct.
    b. Only 1 and 3 are correct.
    c. Only 2 and 4 are correct.
    d. Only 4 is correct.
    e. All are correct.

20. **The principal reason to use high kVp during CT examination is**
    a. better image uniformity.
    b. improved contrast resolution.
    c. improved spatial resolution.
    d. less x-ray tube heat loading.
    e. reduced noise.

21. **Contrast resolution can be improved in CT by**
    1. reducing image noise.
    2. imaging bigger patients.
    3. increasing pixel size.
    4. using high-frequency convolution filter.

    a. Only 1, 2, and 3 are correct.
    b. Only 1 and 3 are correct.
    c. Only 2 and 4 are correct.
    d. Only 4 is correct.
    e. All are correct.

22. **Image CT linearity is best defined as**
    a. a proportional increase in radiation with increasing kVp.
    b. a proportional increase in radiation with increasing mAs.
    c. compensation for artifacts.
    d. not affecting anything.
    e. the ability to assign the correct CT number to a given object.

23. **Good spatial resolution refers to the ability to image**
    a. low spatial frequency objects.
    b. high spatial frequency objects.
    c. small pixels.
    d. low subject contrast tissue.
    e. spatial frequency interfaces.

24. **The term "cupping," as applied in CT, refers to**
    a. an artifact induced by improper beam filtration.
    b. an artifact produced by improper region of interest (ROI).
    c. the appropriate value of Hounsfield unit (HU) in multiple test objects.
    d. the constant value of Hounsfield unit (HU) in a uniform test object.
    e. the decrease in CT number in the middle of a uniform test object.

25. Spatial resolution in CT is improved by
    1. using small detectors.
    2. imaging thick slices.
    3. using small pixel size.
    4. processing with low-frequency convolution.

    a. Only 1, 2, and 3 are correct.
    b. Only 1 and 3 are correct.
    c. Only 2 and 4 are correct.
    d. Only 4 is correct.
    e. All are correct.

26. Computed tomography spatial resolution can be improved by
    1. using a high-frequency reconstruction algorithm.
    2. increasing the number of views required per scan.
    3. reducing the field of view (FOV).
    4. increasing the matrix size.

    a. Only 1, 2, and 3 are correct.
    b. Only 1 and 3 are correct.
    c. Only 2 and 4 are correct.
    d. Only 4 is correct.
    e. All are correct.

27. Which of the following contributes to improved spatial resolution?
    1. small detector size
    2. small pixel size
    3. small voxel size
    4. small patient size

    a. Only 1, 2, and 3 are correct.
    b. Only 1 and 3 are correct.
    c. Only 2 and 4 are correct.
    d. Only 4 is correct.
    e. All are correct.

28. If one wants to improve spatial resolution, which of the following combinations of field of view (FOV) and matrix size would be most effective?
    a. 10 cm FOV, 256^2
    b. 10 cm FOV, 512^2
    c. 15 cm FOV, 512^2
    d. 15 cm FOV, 256^2
    e. 25 cm FOV, 256^2

29. Which type of reconstruction filter would best contribute to improve spatial resolution?
    a. high-frequency convolution filter
    b. low-frequency convolution filter
    c. quadratic convolution filter
    d. ramp convolution filter
    e. step convolution filter

30. **Which of the following are methods for evaluating spatial resolution?**
    1. point spread function
    2. line spread function (LSF)
    3. edge response function (ERF)
    4. ramp spread function

    a. Only 1, 2, and 3 are correct.
    b. Only 1 and 3 are correct.
    c. Only 2 and 4 are correct.
    d. Only 4 is correct.
    e. All are correct.

31. **The spatial resolution of a CT imager can be improved by**
    a. using a smaller x-ray tube.
    b. increasing pixel size.
    c. increasing kVp.
    d. reducing pixel size.
    e. measuring the line spread function (LSF).

32. **Fourier transformation (FT) is a mathematical transformation to convert**
    a. distance into spatial frequency.
    b. distance into time.
    c. point spread function into line spread function (LSF).
    d. spatial frequency into object size.
    e. spatial resolution into contrast resolution.

33. **Image uniformity refers to**
    a. constant CT number of an object.
    b. constant field of view (FOV).
    c. constant patient aperture.
    d. accurate CT numbers.
    e. constant patient dose.

34. **Computed tomography spatial resolution can be improved by**
    1. using a smaller pixel.
    2. thinner slice imaging.
    3. narrowing the predetector collimation.
    4. increasing the source to isocenter distance.

    a. Only 1, 2, and 3 are correct.
    b. Only 1 and 3 are correct.
    c. Only 2 and 4 are correct.
    d. Only 4 is correct.
    e. All are correct.

35. **"Cupping" artifact in a CT image is an example of**
    a. poor contrast resolution.
    b. poor image linearity.
    c. poor image uniformity.
    d. poor spatial resolution.
    e. reconstruction algorithm mismatch.

36. **Fourier transformation (FT) is a method to**
    1. convert an edge response function into a point response function (PRF).
    2. transform object size to spatial frequency.
    3. convert contrast resolution into spatial resolution.
    4. change distance into inverse distance.

    a. Only 1, 2, and 3 are correct.
    b. Only 1 and 3 are correct.
    c. Only 2 and 4 are correct.
    d. Only 4 is correct.
    e. All are correct.

37. **A modulation transfer function (MTF) can be used to estimate spatial resolution**
    a. at high spatial frequencies.
    b. at low spatial frequencies.
    c. at all spatial frequencies.
    d. by converting the point response function (PRF) to an edge response function.
    e. by converting a line spread function to an edge response function (ERF).

38. **Spatial resolution for CT is usually expressed by the**
    a. value of the spatial frequency at a 10% modulation transfer function (MTF).
    b. spatial frequency at an modulation transfer function (MTF) of 1.
    c. spatial frequency at an modulation transfer function (MTF) of 0.
    d. object size at 10% modulation transfer function (MTF).
    e. object size at 0% modulation transfer function (MTF).

39. **At 10 lp/cm the modulation transfer function (MTF) of the pixel is 0.2, that of the collimator assembly 0.12, and that of the detector array 0.23. What is the total modulation transfer function (MTF) for the CT imager?**
    a. 0.006
    b. 0.09
    c. 0.13
    d. 0.36
    e. 0.55

40. **Noise on a CT image principally influences**
    a. contrast resolution.
    b. modulation transfer functioning.
    c. postprocessing functions.
    d. spatial resolution.
    e. the data acquisition system (DAS).

41. **Linearity is particularly important for**
    a. abdomen imaging.
    b. bone mineral measurement.
    c. brain imaging.
    d. cardiac imaging.
    e. maximum intensity projection (MIP).

42. **The principal source of noise in a CT image is**
    a. the data acquisition system (DAS).
    b. improper technique selection.
    c. patient instability.
    d. scatter radiation.
    e. the standard deviation within an region of interest (ROI).

43. **When comparing spiral CT to conventional CT,**
    1. image noise is lower with 180° interpolation in conventional CT.
    2. noise is less with 360° interpolation than 180° interpolation.
    3. transverse resolution is better with spiral CT.
    4. z-axis resolution is better with spiral CT.

    a. Only 1, 2, and 3 are correct.
    b. Only 1 and 3 are correct.
    c. Only 2 and 4 are correct.
    d. Only 4 is correct.
    e. All are correct.

44. **What feature of the CT image is principally limited by increasing image noise?**
    a. artifacts
    b. contrast resolution
    c. imaging uniformity
    d. spatial resolution
    e. z-axis resolution

45. **Contrast resolution can be improved by**
    a. imaging faster.
    b. imaging thicker sections.
    c. using a bone reconstruction filter.
    d. using higher kVp.
    e. a reduced field of view (FOV).

46. **The high contrast region of a contrast-detail curve**
    a. is modulation transfer function (MTF) limited.
    b. is noise limited.
    c. requires image linearity.
    d. requires image uniformity.
    e. should be artifact free.

47. **Spatial resolution is best defined as**
    a. anything that improves image uniformity.
    b. the ability to distinguish low subject contrast tissues.
    c. the ability to image tissue with similar mass density.
    d. the ability to image very small objects.
    e. the ability to reduce image noise.

48. **The principal reason CT exhibits better contrast resolution is**

    a. available postprocessing.
    b. available quantitative analysis.
    c. high kVp imaging.
    d. high mA imaging.
    e. scatter radiation rejection.

49. **Computed tomography image noise can be improved by increasing**

    1. mA.
    2. pixel size.
    3. slice thickness.
    4. kVp.

    a. Only 1, 2, and 3 are correct.
    b. Only 1 and 3 are correct.
    b. Only 2 and 4 are correct.
    d. Only 4 is correct.
    e. All are correct.

50. **Linearity is particularly important for**

    a. bone mineral measurement.
    b. brain imaging.
    c. cardiac imaging.
    d. computed tomography angiography (CTA).
    e. spiral CT.

51. **The value of the modulation transfer function (MTF) at high spatial frequencies is principally related to**

    a. contrast resolution.
    b. spatial resolution.
    c. image noise.
    d. image linearity.
    e. image uniformity.

52. **The Fourier transformation (FT) of a line spread function (LSF) results in**

    a. edge response function (ERF).
    b. modulation transfer function (MTF).
    c. object size.
    d. point response function (PRF).
    e. spatial frequency.

53. **Uniformity in a CT image occurs when**

    a. linear measurements in any direction are accurate.
    b. similar tissue has the same CT number throughout.
    c. the region of interest (ROI) is accurate in all dimensions.
    d. the selected field of view (FOV) is accurate in all dimensions.
    e. various tissues display the appropriate Hounsfield unit (HU).

54. **Spatial resolution in CT is improved by**

    a. imaging low contrast.
    b. using large detectors.
    c. increasing slice thickness.
    d. using small field of view (FOV) and large matrix size.

    a. Only 1, 2, and 3 are correct.
    b. Only 1 and 3 are correct.
    c. Only 2 and 4 are correct.
    d. Only 4 is correct.
    e. All are correct.

55. **Which of the following images should exhibit the highest contrast?**

    a. abdomen
    b. brain
    c. chest
    d. heart
    e. pelvis

56. **Good spatial resolution depends principally on**

    a. pre- and postpatient collimation.
    b. proper kVp.
    c. small pixel size.
    d. thick slice imaging.
    e. type of reconstruction filter.

57. **Contrast resolution is superior with CT examination principally because of**

    a. collimation.
    b. high kVp.
    c. high mA.
    d. postprocessing.
    e. variable slice thickness.

58. **The term "image sharpness" or "image blur" are most closely related to**

    1. artifacts.
    2. image.
    3. contrast resolution.
    4. spatial resolution.

    a. Only 1, 2, and 3 are correct.
    b. Only 1 and 3 are correct.
    c. Only 2 and 4 are correct.
    d. Only 4 is correct.
    e. All are correct.

59. **The low contrast area of a contrast-detail curve**

    a. is modulation transfer function (MTF) limited.
    b. is noise limited.
    c. requires image linearity.
    d. requires image uniformity.
    e. should be artifact free.

60. Contrast resolution can be improved by

    a. imaging faster.
    b. reducing image noise.
    c. using a bone reconstruction filter.
    d. using higher kVp.
    e. a reduced field of view (FOV).

61. Which of the following image characteristics can be obtained from a contrast-detail curve?

    1. spatial resolution
    2. image noise
    3. contrast resolution
    4. linearity

    a. Only 1, 2, and 3 are correct.
    b. Only 1 and 3 are correct.
    c. Only 2 and 4 are correct.
    d. Only 4 is correct.
    e. All are correct.

62. In CT, when going from a 256 × 256 image to a 512 × 512 image, which of the following is true?

    a. resolution decreases, noise decreases, up 2× storage bytes
    b. resolution improves, noise decreases, up 2× storage bytes
    c. resolution improves, noise increases, up 2× storage bytes
    d. resolution improves, noise increases, up 4× storage bytes
    e. resolution improves, noise decreases, up 2× storage bytes

63. The pixel size for a CT body scan with 40-cm field of view (FOV) on a 320 × 320 matrix is

    a. 0.50 mm.
    b. 0.75 mm.
    c. 1.00 mm.
    d. 1.25 mm.
    e. 1.50 mm.

64. A CT scanner has a 512 × 512 matrix over a 25-cm FOV. If the resolution is pixel size limited, the best possible resolution is

    a. 0.5 lp/cm.
    b. 2.5 lp/cm.
    c. 5.0 lp/cm.
    d. 7.5 lp/cm.
    e. 10.0 lp/cm.

65. **In a CT imager**

   1. an 80×80 matrix contains 6400 pixels.
   2. CT numbers are related to the x-ray attenuation coefficient.
   3. the CT number for water is the reference for other materials.
   4. a 256×256 matrix has less resolution than a 160×160 matrix.

   a. Only 1, 2, and 3 are correct.
   b. Only 1 and 3 are correct.
   c. Only 2 and 4 are correct.
   d. Only 4 is correct.
   e. All are correct.

66. **The selection of thin CT slices can affect**

   1. spatial resolution.
   2. quantum mottle.
   3. volume averaging.
   4. CT number.

   a. Only 1, 2, and 3 are correct.
   b. Only 1 and 3 are correct.
   c. Only 2 and 4 are correct.
   d. Only 4 is correct.
   e. All are correct.

67. **The spatial resolution of a CT imager is approximately**

   a. 0.6 lp/mm.
   b. 1 lp/mm.
   c. 3 lp/mm.
   d. 6 lp/mm.
   e. 10 lp/mm.

68. **The visibility of small diagnostically important structures in CT images are likely to increase with increased**

   1. slice thickness.
   2. exposure time at a constant kVp and mAs.
   3. pixel size.
   4. patient dose.

   a. Only 1, 2, and 3 are correct.
   b. Only 1 and 3 are correct.
   c. Only 2 and 4 are correct.
   d. Only 4 is correct.
   e. All are correct.

69. **Assuming that all other factors remain constant, the noise in a CT image will be reduced when**

   1. a slice thickness is increased.
   2. patient thickness is decreased.
   3. mAs is increased.
   4. focal spot size is increased.

a. Only 1, 2, and 3 are correct.
b. Only 1 and 3 are correct.
c. Only 2 and 4 are correct.
d. Only 4 is correct.
e. All are correct.

70. **The contrast resolution of CT is approximately**

a. 0.1%–0.3%.
b. 0.3%–1%.
c. 1%–3%.
d. 3%–10%.
e. 10%–30%.

71. **In regard to CT imagers**

1. spatial resolution is limited by quantum noise.
2. quantum noise can be reduced by increasing scan time.
3. quantum noise will be increased by increasing mA.
4. CT number uniformity can be reduced by beam hardening.

a. Only 1, 2, and 3 are correct.
b. Only 1 and 3 are correct.
c. Only 2 and 4 are correct.
d. Only 4 is correct.
e. All are correct.

72. **Pixel size will have the greatest effect on which CT image property?**

1. CT number
2. noise
3. contrast
4. spatial resolution

a. Only 1, 2, and 3 are correct.
b. Only 1 and 3 are correct.
c. Only 2 and 4 are correct.
d. Only 4 is correct.
e. All are correct.

73. **Linear attenuation coefficient will have the greatest effect on which CT image property?**

1. CT number
2. noise
3. contrast
3. spatial resolution

a. Only 1, 2, and 3 are correct.
b. Only 1 and 3 are correct.
c. Only 2 and 4 are correct.
d. Only 4 is correct.
e. All are correct.

74. Which of the following will increase spatial resolution in a CT image?

    a. increase mA from 200 mA to 500 mA
    b. increase matrix size from 256 × 256 to 512 × 512
    c. increase slice thickness from 5 mm to 10 mm
    d. increase scan time from 2 seconds to 4 seconds
    e. double the gantry rotation speed

75. Which of the following will improve contrast resolution the most in a CT image?

    a. increase mA from 200 mA to 500 mA
    b. increase matrix size from 256 × 256 to 512 × 512
    c. increase slice thickness from 5 mm to 10 mm
    d. increase scan time from 2 seconds to 4 seconds
    e. double the gantry rotation speed

76. Which of the following will change neither spatial nor contrast resolution in a CT image?

    a. increase mA from 200 mA to 500 mA
    b. increase matrix size from 256 × 256 to 512 × 512
    c. increase slice thickness from 5 mm to 10 mm
    d. increase scan time from 2 seconds to 4 seconds
    e. double the gantry rotation speed

77. The CT value of white matter is 40 Hounsfield units (HU). The CT value of gray matter is 45 Hounsfield units (HU). The approximate subject contrast between white and gray matter is

    a. 0.1%.
    b. 0.4%.
    c. 0.45%.
    d. 0.5%.
    e. 5%.

Image Artifacts

- Voluntary and involuntary patient motion can result in a **motion artifact**.

- The motion artifact appears as streaks or step-like patterns at high contrast edges.

- Respiratory motion artifacts in computed tomography angiography (CTA) can simulate vascular stenosis or aneurysm.

- **Metal artifacts** occur because the x-ray absorption results in incomplete projection profiles.

- Metal in tissue gives rise to streak and star-shaped artifacts.

- With penetration of cranial bone, the x-ray beam is selectively filtered and "hardened."

- The hardened x-ray beam presents a false low linear attenuation coefficient and false low CT number.

- The **beam-hardening artifact** appears as a dark ring inside cranial bone and cupping at the center of the image.

- When an object (calcification) is not fully within a slice thickness, the CT number representing that object will be false.

- **Partial volume artifacts** can be reduced by overlapping scans but that increases patient dose.

- Partial volume artifacts can be reduced by using thinner slice thickness but at the expense of higher image noise and/or patient dose.

- Partial volume artifacts can be reduced in spiral CT by moving the plane of reconstruction.

- Multiple reconstruction along the z-axis during spiral CT reduces partial volume artifacts.

- **Ring artifacts** can occur in third-generation CT imagers because of detector malfunction.

- Partial volume artifacts can be reduced by combining several thin slice reconstructed images.

- Pulsation artifact is observed in CTA.

- Pulsation artifact can simulate vascular stenosis.

- Pulsation artifact can be reduced by using 360° interpolation rather than 180° interpolation.

- The **stair-step** artifact is associated with spiral CT.

- The stair-step artifact is most apparent on inclined vessels during spiral CTA.

- The height of a stair step artifact is proportional to couch increment.

- The height of a stair-step artifact is independent of collimation or reconstruction interval.

Chapter 8 Practice Questions

1. **Which of the following are likely to cause a motion artifact on a CT image?**
   1. voluntary patient movement
   2. couch incrementation
   3. involuntary patient motion
   4. gantry rotation

   a. Only 1, 2, and 3 are correct.
   b. Only 1 and 3 are correct.
   c. Only 2 and 4 are correct.
   d. Only 4 is correct.
   e. All are correct.

2. **The best way to correct a partial volume artifact during spiral CT is to**

   a. change the reconstruction plane.
   b. increase pitch.
   c. reduce pitch.
   d. use a thicker slice.
   e. use a thinner slice.

3. **Metal artifacts on a CT image normally appear as**

   a. a herringbone pattern.
   b. cupping.
   c. peaking.
   d. scars.
   e. streaks.

4. **Ring artifacts are best corrected by**

    a. changing slice thickness.
    b. increased matrix size.
    c. proper reconstruction algorithms.
    d. reducing image time.
    e. reducing noise.

5. **The beam-hardening artifact on a CT image appears because of**

    a. x-ray absorption.
    b. cupping.
    c. incorrect linearity.
    d. lack of uniformity.
    e. peaking.

6. **Partial volume artifacts in a CT image appear because of**

    a. detector imbalance.
    b. cupping.
    c. incorrect linearity.
    d. lack of uniformity.
    e. z-axis section position.

7. **The beam-hardening artifact occurs mainly when**

    a. bone is penetrated.
    b. fat is penetrated.
    c. lung tissue is penetrated.
    d. muscle is penetrated.
    e. soft tissue is penetrated.

8. **One manifestation of the beam-hardening artifact is**

    a. high CT number.
    b. increased noise.
    c. loss of contrast resolution.
    d. loss of spatial resolution.
    e. low CT number.

9. **The best way to compensate for motion artifact is to**

    a. change the reconstruction filter.
    b. correct the detector array.
    c. increase matrix size.
    d. recognize the image pattern.
    e. use a thinner slice thickness.

10. **The best way to compensate for a metal artifact is to**

    a. change the reconstruction filter.
    b. correct the detector array.
    c. increase matrix size.
    d. recognize the image pattern.
    e. use a thinner slice thickness.

11. **The best way to compensate for a beam-hardening artifact is to**
    a. change the reconstruction filter.
    b. correct the detector array.
    c. increase matrix size.
    d. recognize the image pattern.
    e. use a thinner slice thickness.

12. **The best way to compensate for a partial volume artifact is to**
    a. recognize the image pattern.
    b. use a thinner slice thickness.
    c. change the reconstruction filter.
    d. correct the detector array.
    e. increase matrix size.

13. **Motion artifacts on a CT image normally appear as**
    a. a herringbone pattern.
    b. cupping.
    c. peaking.
    d. scars.
    e. streaks.

14. **Ring artifacts occur principally in**
    a. first-generation CT imagers.
    b. second-generation CT imagers.
    c. third-generation CT imagers.
    d. fourth-generation CT imagers.
    e. spiral CT.

15. **Artifacts generated by metal implanted in a patient are due to differences in**
    a. absorption characteristics.
    b. beam hardening.
    c. cupping.
    d. imaging time.
    e. peaking.

16. **The "stair-step" artifact is one associated with**
    a. first-generation CT imagers.
    b. second-generation CT imagers.
    c. third-generation CT imagers.
    d. fourth-generation CT imagers.
    e. spiral CT.

17. **The "stair-step" artifact is most bothersome during**
    a. computed tomography angiography (CTA).
    b. quantitative computed tomography (QCT).
    c. CT of the brain.
    d. abdominal CT.
    e. lung CT.

18. Voxel size will effect which CT image characteristic?

    1. spatial resolution
    2. noise
    3. contrast resolution
    4. CT number

    a. Only 1, 2, and 3 are correct.
    b. Only 1 and 3 are correct.
    c. Only 2 and 4 are correct.
    d. Only 4 is correct.
    e. All are correct.

19. **Partial volume artifacts in CT are**

    a. reduced when the beam width is increased.
    b. reduced when scan time is increased.
    c. increased by the heterogeneity of the tissue within a voxel.
    d. increased with added filtration.
    e. not visible in fourth-generation scanners.

20. **Ring artifacts in third-generation CT scanners are usually due to**

    a. kVp shift during the scan.
    b. tube arching.
    c. detector calibration drift.
    d. beam hardening.
    e. patient motion.

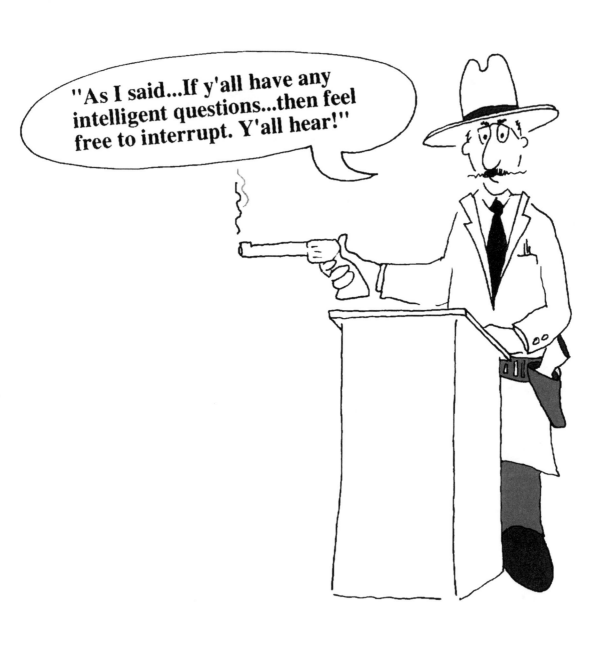

Radiation Safety

PATIENT RADIATION DOSE

- Generally, patient radiation dose is higher during computed tomography (CT) than during radiography or fluoroscopy.

- Patient radiation dose during CT is approximately 5000 mrad per examination.

- Patient radiation dose during radiography is approximately 5 mrad/mAs or 100 mrad per examination.

- Patient radiation dose during spiral CT is rather independent of collimation.

- Patient radiation dose during fluoroscopy is approximately 4000 mrad/min, with doses ranging from 1000–100,000 mrad per examination.

- Patient radiation dose during spiral CT is inversely proportional to pitch.

- Patient radiation dose during CT is nearly uniform throughout the body, while that from radiography or fluoroscopy is maximum at the entrance skin.

- For a given collimation during spiral CT, higher pitch results in lower patient radiation dose.

- Patient radiation dose is often less in spiral CT because overlapping images can be reconstructed without overlapping scans.

- Patient radiation dose during CT is higher with thinner slices or overlapping slices.

- As with any x-ray imaging, patient dose can be reduced at the expense of image noise.

patient dose is increased with:
- repeat scan
- low pitch
- thin slices
- overlapping slices

approximate patient dose

	Tissue dose (mrad)	Effective dose (mrem)
Head		
-newborn	4100	600
-child	3900	300
-adult	3700	150
Abdomen		
-newborn	2000	500
-child	1400	400
-adult	1100	300

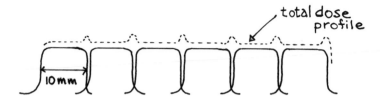

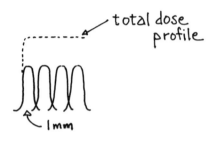

$$mSAD = CTDI\left(\frac{ST}{CI}\right)$$

- When patient dose is specified for a CT examination, it is usually an average value of a dose distribution.

- The dose profile is most helpful in identifying patient dose.

- Patient dose in CT is measured with a pencil ionization chamber.

- Patient dose in CT is described by the CT dose index (CTDI).

- The CTDI is equal to the multiple scan average dose (MSAD) if the slice thickness (ST) is equal to the couch incrementation (CI).

- If the ST does not equal CI, MSAD is equal to the CTDI multiplied by CI.

PERSONNEL RADIATION EXPOSURE

- Area radiation exposure is figure-eight shaped.

- Lowest area radiation exposures are in the plane of the gantry and outside the patient aperture.

- Highest area radiation exposure is near the patient and is due to scatter radiation produced in the patient.

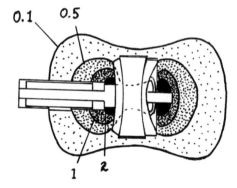

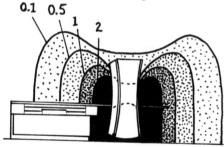

mR/scan

ALARA:
- minimize time
- maximize distance
- use shielding

- Area radiation exposure is approximately 1 mR/scan at 1 m from the scan plane.

- It is permissible for a CT technologist to remain in the room during examination but protective apparel must be worn.

- When a technologist is in the room during examination, the radiation monitor should be positioned at collar level above the protective apron.

- Always practice As Low As Reasonably Achievable (ALARA) by applying the Cardinal Principles of Radiation Protection—time, distance, shielding.

CONTRAST MEDIA

- The number of particles of contrast media (solute) per kg of water (solvent) is **osmolity**.

- High osmolity contrast media (HOCM) is the conventional "ionic" contrast media.

- Blood has an osmolity of approximately 300 mOsm/kg water.

- High osmolity contrast media has 4 to 8 times the osmolity of blood (1200 to 2500 mOsm/kg).

- High osmolity contrast media is considered to be more toxic than low osmolity contrast media (LOCM).

- Low osmolity contrast media is "nonionic" contrast media.

- Low osmolity contrast media has 2 to 3 times the osmolity of blood (600−800 mOsm/kg water).

- Contrast media has a biologic half-life of 10 to 90 min.

- Ninety percent of contrast media is excreted within 24 hours.

- Peak urine concentration occurs approximately 2 hours following administration.

- Contrast media can be excreted through liver but the principal clearance route is kidney.

- Patients with poor renal function have increased excretion of contrast media through gallbladder and small intestine.

- Contrast media does not change when excreted in mother's milk.

- Contrast media enhances contrast resolution by increased photoelectric effect.

- Atomic number for iodine is 53 (Z:53).

- Degree of contrast enhancement is directly related to iodine concentration.

- Following intravenous (IV) injection, peak iodine blood concentration occurs within 2 min.

- Following IV injection, the vascular compartment biologic half-life for iodinated contrast is approximately 20 min.

Approximate CTDI (120 kVp, 340 mAs, 10 mm)

Head
  surface   4000 mrad
  center   4000 mrad

Body
  surface   2000 mrad
  center   1000 mrad

mOsm/kg = milliosmoles per kilogram

post injection reaction time
  <5 min (70%)
  5-15 min (15%)
  >15 min (15%)

IV contrast

	Injection Rate (ml/s)	Amount(ml)	Delay scan(s)
Head and neck	1.5	120	40
Chest	1.5	75	30-40
Abdominal vessels	1.5-2	120-150	60-70

- Iodinated contrast media is transferred from the vascular to the extravascular compartment in about 10 min for equilibrium followed by an exponential decrease in both.

- Renal accumulation occurs in approximately 1 min with maximum contrast occurring in 5 to 15 min.

- Severely impaired renal function results in prolonged plasma levels and poor contrast resolution.

- Contrast media should be warmed to body temperature before administration.

- Contrast media may be administered by bolus injection or rapid infusion.

- Adult dosage is 150 ml to 250 ml.

- Child dosage is 1 ml/kg to 3 ml/kg.

- Less contrast media is required for spiral CT.

- An over dosage may be life threatening by compromising the cardiovascular or pulmonary systems.

- Contrast media is dialyzable since it does not bind to plasma or serum protein.

- Reaction to contrast media is unpredictable. Personnel must be trained to recognize contrast media reaction and respond appropriately.

- Fatal contrast media reactions reportedly occur from 6 to 100/M.

contraindications for contrast media:
- previous reaction
- asthma/hay fever
- liver or kidney dysfunction
- diabetic
- pregnant
- multiple studies scheduled

Chapter 9 Practice Questions

1. Which of the following is likely to result in highest patient dose?

   a. CT
   b. chest radiography
   c. intravenous pyleography (IVP)
   d. barium enema
   e. portable radiography

2. The adult dosage of contrast media for a CT examination is the range of

   a. 1–15 ml.
   b. 15–50 ml.
   c. 50–150 ml.
   d. 150–250 ml.
   e. 250–1000 ml.

3. If one increases the pitch during spiral CT,

   1. patient dose is reduced.
   2. transverse resolution is reduced.
   3. axial resolution is reduced.
   4. contrast resolution is reduced.

   a. Only 1, 2, and 3 are correct.
   b. Only 1 and 3 are correct.
   c. Only 2 and 4 are correct.
   d. Only 4 is correct.
   e. All are correct.

4. Which of the following are contraindications for contrast media administration?

   1. a previous reaction
   2. asthma
   3. hay fever
   4. liver dysfunction

   a. Only 1, 2, and 3 are correct.
   b. Only 1 and 3 are correct.
   c. Only 2 and 4 are correct.
   d. Only 4 is correct.
   e. All are correct.

5. Lowest occupational radiation exposure during a CT examination is

   a. in the plane of the gantry.
   b. at the imaging plane.
   c. at the head of the patient.
   d. at the foot of the patient.
   e. at the operating console group.

6. Characteristics of conventional ionic contrast include

   a. high osmolity.
   b. low osmolity.
   c. extended injection rate.
   d. increased injection volume.
   e. water concentration.

7. Which of the following is the approximate patient dose during a CT examination?

   a. 1000 mrad (10 mGy$_t$)
   b. 5000 mrad (50 mGy$_t$)
   c. 10,000 mrad (100 mGy$_t$)
   d. 15,000 mrad (150 mGy$_t$)
   e. 25,000 mrad (250 mGy$_t$)

8. Contrast media administered for CT examination is principally removed from the body through the

   a. kidney.
   b. liver.
   c. lung.
   d. colon.
   e. esophagus.

9. During CT examination with the technologist in the control booth, the occupational radiation monitor should be positioned

   a. anywhere on the trunk of the body.
   b. at waist level.
   c. at chest level.
   d. at collar level.
   e. on the dominant hand.

10. The principal reason that contrast media will increase contrast resolution of a CT image is

    a. Compton scatter.
    b. photoelectric absorption.
    c. coherent scatter.
    d. pair production.
    e. bremsstrahlung.

11. Which of the following are contraindications for contrast media administration?

    1. kidney dysfunction
    2. diabetes
    3. pregnancy
    4. multiple studies scheduled

    a. Only 1, 2, and 3 are correct.
    b. Only 1 and 3 are correct.
    c. Only 2 and 4 are correct.
    d. Only 4 is correct.
    e. All are correct.

12. During CT examination of the abdomen, the patient effective dose (E) will be closest to

    a. 100 mrem (1 mSv).
    b. 500 mrem (5 mSv).
    c. 1000 mrem (10 mSv).
    d. 5000 mrem (50 mSv).
    e. 10,000 mrem (100 mSv).

13. The dosage of contrast media for pediatric CT imaging is approximately

    a. 1–3 ml/kg.
    b. 3–6 ml/kg.
    c. 6–10 ml/kg.
    d. 10–20 ml/kg.
    e. 20–50 ml/kg.

14. During CT examination, the radiologic technologist should observe the principles of **As Low As Reasonably Achievable (ALARA)**, which include

    1. minimize time in the examination room.
    2. increase distance from the radiation source.
    3. use protective shielding where appropriate.
    4. position radiation monitor at collar level.

    a. Only 1, 2, and 3 are correct.
    b. Only 1 and 3 are correct.
    c. Only 2 and 4 are correct.
    d. Only 4 is correct.
    e. All are correct.

15. Osmolity is a term that refers to

    a. the concentration of contrast media particles.
    b. the duration of contrast injection.
    c. the duration of contrast retention.
    d. injection rate.
    e. the concentration of water.

16. A good rule of thumb for area radiation exposure during CT examination is

    a. 1 mR per scan at 1 m from the patient.
    b. 10 mR per scan at 1 m from the patient.
    c. 100 mR per scan at 1 m from the patient.
    d. 1 mR per scan at the operating console.
    e. 1 mR per scan outside the room.

17. The characteristics of nonionic contrast media include

    a. high osmolity.
    b. low osmolity.
    c. extended injection rate.
    d. increased injection volume.
    e. water concentration.

18. During CT examination, the technologist

    a. may remain in the room but should wear protective apparel.
    b. may remain in the room and protective apparel is unnecessary.
    c. may not enter the room.
    d. must remain in the control booth area.
    e. must remain in the control booth area with protective apparel.

19. If a contrast reaction is to occur, it will likely occur within

    a. 5 min.
    b. 5–15 min.
    c. 15–30 min.
    d. 30 min–1 hour.
    e. 1–3 hours.

20. During CT imaging, if the technologist is in the imaging room, the occupational radiation monitor should be positioned

    a. anywhere on the trunk of the body.
    b. at waist level.
    c. at chest level.
    d. at collar level.
    e. on the dominant hand.

21. Patient radiation dose increases with

    1. thinner slices.
    2. lower pitch.
    3. overlapping slices.
    4. larger image matrix.

    a. Only 1, 2, and 3 are correct.
    b. Only 1 and 3 are correct.
    c. Only 2 and 4 are correct.
    d. Only 4 is correct.
    e. All are correct.

22. During CT examination of the abdomen, the approximate entrance skin exposure will be closest to

    a. 100 mR (1 mGy$_a$).
    b. 500 mR (5 mGy$_a$).
    c. 1000 mR (10 mGy$_a$).
    d. 5000 mR (50 mGy$_a$).
    e. 10,000 mR (100 mGy$_a$).

23. Occupational radiation exposure during CT imaging is principally due to

    a. scatter from the patient.
    b. leakage from the x-ray tube.
    c. useful beam penetration.
    d. scatter from the gantry.
    e. scatter from the wall of the examination room.

24. During CT examination of the abdomen, the approximate CT dose index (CTDI) will be

    a. 100 mrad (1 mGy$_t$).
    b. 500 mrad (5 mGy$_t$).
    c. 1000 mrad (10 mGy$_t$).
    d. 5000 mrad (50 mGy$_t$).
    e. 10,000 mrad (100 mGy$_t$).

Quality Control

CHAPTER
10

- The CT number of water should be zero.

- Scan a water phantom, select a large enough region of interest (ROI), the average CT number should be within ±3.

- Scan an empty gantry aperture, select a large ROI, the average CT number for air should be within −1000±5.

- Computed tomography (CT) noise is evaluated by scanning a water bath. The standard deviation (σ) should not exceed ±10.

- Spatial resolution is evaluated by scanning any number of phantoms-hole patterns, or line pair patterns.

- Spatial resolution should be at least equal to the manufacturer's specifications.

- Most CT imagers can image 0.5 mm (10 lp/cm), some as good as 0.2 mm (20 lp/cm) in a high resolution mode.

- Contrast resolution is evaluated with either a phantom, thick or thin, various hole sizes filled with water, or various hole sizes of various depth for partial volume effects.

- Contrast resolution should be at least 5 mm at 5% contrast.

- Distance measurement accuracy is evaluated by imaging the American Association of Physicists in Medicine (AAPM) test object that has pins separated by 10 mm.

- The electronic distance calipers must be accurate to within ±5%.

- The video monitor should be evaluated for distortion by pressing a clear plastic ruler against the screen image of the 10 mm pin test object to ensure the same 5% accuracy.

141

- Scan plane localization, usually a laser light localizer, should be accurate to within 1 mm. A number of test devices are available.

- Patient couch indexing can be checked with cardboard wrapped film or marks on the couch and rail. The limit of error is 1%.

- Slice width is usually evaluated with a ramp test object and should be within 50% for nominal widths of 5 mm and above and 100% for thinner slices.

Chapter 10 Practice Questions

1. When scanning a water bath, the resulting value in Hounsfield units (HU) should be

   a. −1000.
   b. −50.
   c. 0.
   d. 50.
   e. +1000.

2. A spiral CT examination is programmed to travel 240 mm of the patient anatomy, the final position of the patient couch should be within

   a. 239–241 mm.
   b. 238–242 mm.
   c. 235–245 mm.
   d. 230–250 mm.
   e. 225–255 mm.

3. When operated in the high resolution mode, a good CT imager will have spatial resolution of approximately

   a. 0.1 mm.
   b. 0.2 mm.
   c. 0.5 mm.
   d. 1.0 mm.
   e. 2.0 mm.

4. When evaluated by imaging a test object, electronic calipers should be accurate to within

   a. ±1%.
   b. ±5%.
   c. ±10%.
   d. ±20%.
   e. ±25%.

5. Computed tomography image noise is evaluated by the

   a. accuracy of Hounsfield units (HU) for various materials.
   b. accuracy of linear measurement.
   c. accuracy of the area of a region of interest (ROI).
   d. standard deviation of a water bath image.
   e. standard deviation of an air scan.

6. The best way to evaluate noise in a CT image is to scan

   a. a line pair phantom.
   b. a star phantom.
   c. a water bath.
   d. air.
   e. the AAPM 5-pin insert.

7. When a test object is positioned outside of the scan plane using the laser light localizer, then moved to the scan plane, the new position should be how close to the scan plane?

   a. within 1 mm
   b. within 2 mm
   c. within 5 mm
   d. within 10 mm
   e. within 20 mm

8. An appropriate value of spatial resolution for a CT imager operated in the normal mode is approximately

   a. 0.1 mm.
   b. 0.2 mm.
   c. 0.5 mm.
   d. 1.0 mm.
   e. 2.0 mm.

9. The amount of error allowed in the movement of the patient couch when expressed as a percentage of the total intended movement is

   a. $\pm 1\%$.
   b. $\pm 2\%$.
   c. $\pm 5\%$.
   d. $\pm 10\%$.
   e. $\pm 20\%$.

10. When operated in the high resolution mode, a good CT imager will have spatial resolution of approximately

    a. 1 lp/cm.
    b. 2 lp/cm.
    c. 5 lp/cm.
    d. 10 lp/cm.
    e. 20 lp/cm.

11. An object has Hounsfield units (HU) of 50 and the surrounding tissue of 500, the contrast is

    a. 0.5%.
    b. 1%.
    c. 5%.
    d. 10%.
    e. 50%.

12. Contrast resolution is best evaluated imaging a test object

    a. designed for partial volume effects.
    b. filled with water.
    c. filled with air.
    d. of the AAPM 5-pin insert.
    e. of a line pair phantom.

13. Which of the following is normally used to evaluate contrast resolution?

    1. a water-filled phantom containing a pane of plastic with various size holes
    2. a water-filled phantom
    3. a plastic phantom with holes of various sizes and various depths
    4. a line pair phantom

    a. Only 1, 2, and 3 are correct.
    b. Only 1 and 3 are correct.
    c. Only 2 and 4 are correct.
    d. Only 4 is correct.
    e. All are correct.

14. Acceptable contrast resolution occurs when a CT imager can display an object of at least

    a. 5 mm at 5% contrast.
    b. 5 mm at 10% contrast.
    c. 10 mm at 5% contrast.
    d. 10 mm at 10% contrast.
    e. 10 mm at 20% contrast.

15. When operating in the normal mode, a good CT imager will have spatial resolution of approximately

    a. 1 lp/cm.
    b. 2 lp/cm.
    c. 5 lp/cm.
    d. 10 lp/cm.
    e. 20 lp/cm.

16. Electronic distance calipers used for image analysis during postprocessing are best evaluated with

    a. a line pair phantom.
    b. a water bath.
    c. a region of interest (ROI) phantom.
    d. the AAPM 5-pin test object.
    e. the AAPM test object having multiple pins separated by 10 mm.

17. When scanning an empty gantry (air scan) and selecting a large region of interest (ROI), the standard deviation should not exceed

    a. ± 1 HU.
    b. ± 3 HU.
    c. ± 5 HU.
    d. ± 10 HU.
    e. ± 20 HU.

18. The laser light localization of the scan plane should be accurate to within

    a. 1 mm.
    b. 2 mm.
    c. 5 mm.
    d. $\pm 2\%$ of the SID.
    e. $\pm 5\%$ of the SID.

19. Spatial resolution in a CT imager is best evaluated by scanning

    a. a water bath.
    b. air.
    c. the AAPM 5-pin insert.
    d. a star test object.
    e. a line pair test object.

20. The patient is moved 10 times at 10 mm each (100 mm), the final position of the couch should be between

    a. 99 and 101 mm.
    b. 98 and 102 mm.
    c. 95 and 105 mm.
    d. 90 and 110 mm.
    e. 80 and 120 mm.

21. When scanning an empty gantry aperture (air scan), the resulting Hounsfield unit (HU) should be

    a. -1000.
    b. -50.
    c. 0.
    d. 50.
    e. $+1000$.

22. When analyzing the results of a water bath scan using a large region of interest (ROI), the standard deviation of results should be within

    a. ± 1 HU.
    b. ± 3 HU.
    c. ± 5 HU.
    d. ± 10 HU.
    e. ± 20 HU.

23. Slice thickness is normally evaluated with

    a. a line pair phantom.
    b. a partial volume phantom test object.
    c. a test object containing a ramp.
    d. the AAPM 10 mm multiple pin insert.
    e. the AAPM 5-pin insert.

Appendices

Glossary

Absolute risk Incidence of malignant disease in a population each 1 year following a given dose. Expressed as number of cases/10^6 persons/rem.

Absorbed dose Energy transferred from ionizing radiation per unit mass of irradiated material. Expressed in rad (100 erg/g) or gray (1 J/kg).

Absorber Any material that absorbs or reduces the intensity of radiation.

Absorption Transfer of energy from radiation to matter. Removal of x-rays from a beam via the photoelectric effect.

Acute Beginning suddenly and running a short but rather severe course.

Acute effects (See Early effects).

Added filtration Aluminum (or its equivalent) of appropriate thickness positioned outside an x-ray tube and in the primary beam.

ALARA The principle that radiation exposure should be kept as low as reasonably achievable, economic and social factors being taken into account.

Algorithm Computer-adapted mathematical calculation applied to raw data during the process of image reconstruction. Computer-compatible equation.

Aliasing Effect Artifacts that appear on the CT image as fine lines. They occur when too few samples are acquired. Also called sampling artifacts.

Aluminum (Al) Metal most frequently selected as x-ray beam filter material because it effectively removes low-energy x-rays.

Aluminum equivalent Thickness of a material resulting in the same attenuation as aluminum.

American Association of Physicists in Medicine (AAPM) Scientific society of medical physicists.

American College of Medical Physicists (ACMP) Professional society of medical physicists.

American College of Radiology (ACR) Professional society of radiologists and medical physicists.

American Society of Radiologic Technologists (ASRT) Scientific and professional society of radiographers.

Ampere (A) The SI unit of electric charge. 1 A = 1 C/s.

Analog signal Continuous display of energy, intensity, or radiation, as opposed to the discrete display of a digital signal.

Anode Positive side of x-ray tube, containing the target.

Anthropomorphic human characteristics.

Aperture a. Circular opening for the patient in the gantry of a CT or magnetic resonance imager. b. Fixed collimation of a diagnostic x-ray tube as in an aperture diaphragm. c. Variable opening before the lens of a cine- or photospot camera.

Archival storage Secondary or permanent storage of digital images—usually magnetic tapes, magnetic disks, or optical disks—and film images.

Archiving Saving data on auxiliary devices, such as optical disk or digital audiotape, for the purpose of reviewing at a later date.

Area beam X-ray beam pattern usually shaped as a square or rectangle used in conventional radiography and fluoroscopy.

Array processor Part of a computer that accepts signal data and performs the mathematical calculations necessary to reconstruct a digital image.

Artifact Pattern on an image that does not represent anatomy and does not exist in reality. It may be caused by operator error, patient motion or equipment characteristics. Unintended optical density on a radiograph or other film-type image receptor.

Attenuation Reduction in radiation intensity when passing through matter as a result of absorption and scattering.

Attenuation coefficient Numerical expression of the decrease in intensity with penetration into matter. Process of energy absorption, described by percent of radiation remaining after x-rays pass through an object. The x-ray attenuation coefficient is expressed in inverse length (m^{-1}, cm^{-1}).

Attenuation profile Result of the CT process that accounts for the attenuation properties of each ray sum relative to the position of the ray.

Attenuator Device or material that reduces x-ray or ultrasound intensity.

Axial Parallel to the long axis of the body.

Axial Plane Imaginary plane that divides the body into right and left or front and back sections-sagittal or coronal, respectively.

Back Projection Process of converting the data from the attenuation profile to a matrix.

Backscatter X-rays that have interacted with an object and are deflected in a backward direction.

Beam Hardening Artifact Artifact that results from lower-energy photons being preferentially absorbed, leaving higher-energy photons to strike the detector array.

Bolus Phase Phase of contrast enhancement that immediately follows an intravenous bolus injection. Characterized by an attenuation difference of 30 or more Hounsfield units between the aorta and the inferior vena cava.

Bremsstrahlung X-rays produced by deceleration of electrons near the nucleus of a target atom; braking radiation.

Calibration Comparison of a laboratory source or instrument in daily use with a standard source or instrument to improve accuracy.

Carcinogenic Causing cancer.

Cataractogenic Causing cataracts.

Cataracts Clouding of the lens resulting in vision obstruction.

Cathode Negative side of the x-ray tube, contains the filament and focusing cup.

Cathode ray tube (CRT) Electron beam vacuum tube designed for a two-dimensional display. A TV picture tube used to display CT image and to communicate with computer.

Center for Devices and Radiological Health (CDRH) Agency of the U.S. Food and Drug Administration. Responsible for a national radiation control program.

Centigray 0.01 Gy. (1 rad)

Central Processing Unit (CPU) Primary component of a computer. The CPU takes information from the data acquisition system and manipulates it so that an image can be formed.

Characteristic x-rays X-rays produced following ionization of inner-shell electrons of the target element.

Charged particle An ion. Elementary particle carrying a positive or negative electric charge.

Classical scattering Scattering of x-rays with no loss of energy. Also called **coherent, Rayleigh,** or **Thompson scattering.**

Coherent scattering (See Classical scattering.)

Collimation Restriction of the useful x-ray beam to the anatomical area of interest in order to reduce patient dose and improve image contrast.

Compensating filter Material inserted between an x-ray source and a patient to shape the intensity of the x-ray beam. X-ray beam filter designed to make the remnant beam more uniform in intensity, such as a bow tie filter.

Compton effect Interaction between an x-ray and a loosely bound outer-shell electron, resulting in ionization and x-ray scattering.

Compton electron Electron emitted from the outer shell of an atom as a result of x-ray interaction.

Computed tomography (CT) Creation of a transverse tomographic section of the body using a rotating fan beam, detector array, and computed reconstruction.

Computerized axial tomography (CAT) Early term used to describe CT imaging. Since images produced are taken at various angles, "axial" has been deleted.

Conduction Transfer of heat by molecular agitation.

Conductor Material that allows heat or electric current to flow relatively easily.

Contrast Range of shades of gray on an image.

Contrast resolution Ability to detect, image and display similar tissues such as gray-white matter and liver-spleen.

Control badge Personnel radiation monitor provided with each batch of badges to allow determination of exposure while in transit.

Control chart Graphical plot of quality control test results with respect to time or sequence of measurement along with acceptance limits.

Control limits Limits shown on a control chart beyond which performance is compromised and corrective action required.

Controlled area Area where personnel occupancy and activity are subject to control and supervision for the purpose of radiation protection. Such personnel usually wear personnel radiation monitors.

Convection Transfer of heat by the movement of hot air or water to a colder place.

Convolution Process of applying a mathematic formula (filter function) to an attenuation profile.

Coolidge tube The type of vacuum tube in use today allows x-ray intensity and energy to be separately and accurately selected.

Coronal plane Imaginary plane that divides the body into anterior and posterior sections.

Coulomb (C) SI unit of electric charge.

Coulomb per kilogram (C/kg) SI unit of radiation exposure. $2.58 = 10^{-4}$ C/kg = 1 R.

CRT (See Cathode ray tube.)

CT numbers Numbers used to define relative attenuation coefficient for each pixel of tissue in image as compared with attenuation coefficient of water.

Cupping Artifact Artifact that results from beam hardening. It appears on the image as a vague area of increased optical density in a somewhat concentric shape around the periphery of an image, similar to the shape of a cup.

Cursor Electronic pointer used to outline areas of interest on a digital image for analysis. Used to highlight all the pixels of an area.

Data Acquisition System Component following the CT detector array that samples each detector and transmits the signal to the computer. It is located on the gantry.

Densitometer Device that measures optical density.

Detector Device that is sensitive to x-rays and can measure x-ray intensity.

Detector array Group of detectors and the interspace material used to separate them. The image receptor in CT.

Detector Efficiency Ability of the detector to capture transmitted x-rays and change them to electronic signals.

Diagnostic-type protective tube housing Lead-lined housing enclosing an x-ray tube that shields leakage radiation to less than 100 mR/h at 1 m.

Diaphragm Device that restricts an x-ray beam to a fixed size.

Differential absorption Varying degrees of absorption in different tissues that results in image contrast and formation of an x-ray image.

Diode Vacuum tube with two electrodes.

Direct current Flow of electricity in only one direction in a conductor.

Display Field of View Determines how much of the raw data is used to display an image. Also called zoom, or target view.

Dose Amount of energy absorbed by an irradiated object per unit mass. Expressed in rad or gray (Gy).

Dose equivalent (H) Radiation quantity used for radiation protection purposes that expresses dose on a common scale for all radiations. Expressed in rem or sievert (Sv).

Dosimeter Instrument for detecting and measuring exposure to ionizing radiation.

Dosimetry Theory and application of principles and techniques involved in the measurement and recording of radiation dose. Quantitative determination of spatial and temporal radiation exposure.

Dynamic range Range of values that can be displayed by an imaging system; shades of gray.

Dynamic Scanning Process by which scans are acquired quickly, often after a rapid bolus injection of intravenous contrast material.

Early effects Effects of ionizing radiation that appear within weeks of exposure. Also called **acute effects**.

Edge Gradient Effect Straight line artifacts that radiate from a high-contrast area, such as bone and soft tissue.

Effective atomic number Weighted average atomic number of tissue.

Effective dose (E) Sum over specified tissues of the products of the equivalent dose in a tissue (H_T) and the weighting factor for that tissue (W_T) (i.e., $E = \Sigma W_T H_T$).

Effective Slice Thickness Thickness of the slice that is actually represented on the CT image, as opposed to the size selected by the collimator opening. Because of the interpolation process used in spiral CT, the effective slice thickness may be wider than the selected slice thickness.

Electromagnetic radiation X-rays, γ-rays, and some nonionizing radiation such as ultraviolet, infrared, and radiowaves. Oscillating electric and magnetic fields that travel in a vacuum with the velocity of light.

Electromagnetic spectrum Continuum of electromagnetic radiation.

Electrometer Device used to measure elecric charge.

Electromotive force Electric potential. Expressed in volts (V).

Electron Elementary particle with one negative charge. Electrons surround the positively charged nucleus and determine the chemical properties of an atom.

Electron volt (eV) Unit of energy equal to that which an electron acquires from a potential difference of 1 V.

Energy Ability to do work. Expressed in joule (J).

Entrance skin exposure (ESE) X-ray exposure of the skin. Expressed in mR or air kerma Gy_a.

Equilibrium Phase Last phase of contrast enhancement. Occurs when the attenuation difference between the aorta and the inferior vena cava is less than 10 Hounsfield units.

Error Difference between the measured value and the true value of a parameter or a quantity.

Exponent Superscript or power to which ten is raised in scientific notation.

Exposure Measure of the ionization produced in air by x- or γ-rays. Amount of ionizing radiation incident on tissue. Expressed in R, C/kg, or air kerma Gy_a.

Extravasation Seepage of intravenous solution into surrounding soft tissue.

Fan beam X-ray beam pattern used in CT; projected as a slit.

Filament That part of the cathode that emits electrons resulting in x-ray tube current.

Film badge Most widely used type of personnel radiation monitor. Pack of photographic film used for measurement of radiation exposure to radiation workers.

Filter Added material that increases effective x-ray energy by absorbing low-energy x-rays. Device designed to reduce patient dose.

Filtration Removal of low-energy x-rays from the useful beam with aluminum or other metal. Results in increased beam quality and reduced patient dose.

Floppy Disk A flexible plastic disk coated with magnetic material used to store computer data.

Focal spot Area of the anode where electrons interact to produce x-rays; the target.

Focusing cup Metal shroud surrounding the filament.

Force That which changes the motion of an object. A push or pull. Expressed in newtons (N).

Gantry Framework that holds x-ray tube and radiation detection system. Portion of the CT or magnetic resonance imager that accommodates the patient and source and detector assemblies.

Geometric Efficiency Fraction of the actual detector area intercepting the x-ray beam. That not included is interspace.

Gonadal shield Device used during radiologic procedures to protect the reproductive organs from exposure to the useful beam when they are in or within about 5 cm of a collimated beam.

Gray (Gy) Special name for the SI unit of absorbed dose and air kerma. 1 Gy = 1 J/kg = 100 rad.

Gray Scale System that assigns a given number of Hounsfield values to each level of gray determined by the window width.

Half-Scan Scan produced from an x-ray tube arc typically acquired from 180°. Also called partial scan.

Half-value layer (HVL) Thickness of absorber necessary to reduce an x-ray beam to half its original intensity.

Hard copy Permanent image on film or paper, as opposed to an image on CRT, disk, or magnetic tape.

Health physics Science concerned with recognition, evaluation and control of radiation hazards.

Heat Dissipation Ability of the x-ray tube to rid itself of heat.

Heel effect Absorption of x-rays in the heel of the target, resulting in reduced x-ray intensity to the anode side of the central axis.

Helical Scanning (See Spiral CT.)

Hertz (Hz) Unit of frequency; wavelengths cycles or oscillations per second of a simple harmonic motion.

High-contrast resolution Ability to image small objects having high subject contrast; spatial resolution.

High-pass filter Convolution filter that suppresses the resolution of low-contrast tissue (liver/spleen) and enhances the resolution of high-contrast tissue (bone edges).

Histogram Display function that creates a bar graph to show the range of CT numbers within a specified region of interest.

Hounsfield unit (HU) Scale of CT numbers used to judge the nature of tissue. Also called pixel values, or CT numbers.

Image Magnification Postprocessing method of increasing the image size as it appears on the monitor.

Image Processor Component of a CT system that converts digitized data to shades of gray to be displayed on a cathode-ray tube monitor.

Image Reconstruction Use of raw data to create a CT image.

Inherent filtration Filtration of useful x-ray beam provided by the permanently installed components of an x-ray tube housing assembly and the glass window of the x-ray tube.

International System of Units (SI) Standard system of units based on the meter, kilogram, and second adopted by all countries and used in all branches of science.

Inverse square law Law stating that the intensity of radiation at a location is inversely proportional to the square of its distance from the source of radiation.

Ion Atom with too many or too few electrons, or a free electron; electrically charged particle.

Ion pair Two oppositely charged particles usually a positively charged atom and an electron.

Ionic/Nonionic Characteristic of intravenous iodinated contrast medium that relates to its chemical composition. Ionic refers to a type that forms ions in water solution. Nonionic contrast medium does not dissociate and therefore does not ionize in water.

Ionization Removal of an electron from an atom.

Ionizing radiation Radiation capable of ionization.

Isotonic Having nearly the same number of particles in solution as water.

Joule (J) Unit of energy. The work done when a force of 1 N acts on an object along a distance of 1 m.

Kerma (k) Energy absorbed per unit mass from the initial Kinetic Energy Released in Matter of all the electrons liberated by x- or γ-rays. Expressed in gray (Gy). 1 Gy = 1 J/kg. Gy_a = air kerma. Gy_t = tissue dose.

Kiloelectron volt (keV) Energy equal to 1,000 eV.

Kilogram (kg) 1,000 g.

Kilovolt (kV) Measure of the high voltage produced by the x-ray generator. Qualitative measure of the x-ray beam. Electrical potential equal to 1,000 V.

Kinetic energy Energy of motion.

Late effects Effects that appear months or years after exposure to ionizing radiation.

Lead equivalent Thickness of radiation-absorbing material that produces an attenuation equivalent to that produced by a specified amount of lead.

Leakage radiation Secondary radiation emitted through the x-ray tube housing, not including the useful beam.

Linear energy transfer (LET) Measure of the ability of energy transfer to biological material. Expressed in keV/μm of soft tissue.

Low-contrast resolution Ability to image objects with similar subject contrast.

Low-pass filter Mathematical filter that suppresses the resolution of high-frequency structures (bone edges) and enhances the resolution of low-frequency structures (liver/spleen or gray/white matter).

Magnetic tape Data storage device that consists of large reels of tape.

mAs (See Milliampere seconds).

Mass Quantity of matter (measured in kg).

Matrix Array of numbers in rows and columns of pixels displayed on a digital image. e.g. 256 × 256, 320 × 320, or 512 × 512.

Matter Anything that occupies space and has form or shape.

Mean energy Average energy of an x-ray beam.

Mega- Prefix that multiplies a basic unit by 1,000,000 or 10^6.

Micro- Prefix that divides a basic unit into 1 million parts or 10^{-6}.

Milli- Prefix that divides a basic unit by 1,000 or 10^{-3}.

Milliampere (mA) Measure of x-ray tube current used in the production of x-rays. Coupled with the imaging time, it is the quantitative measure of the x-ray beam.

Milliampere seconds (mAs) Product of exposure time and x-ray tube current. A measure of the total number of electrons, used to produce the x-ray beam.

Misregistration Misalignment of two or more images because of patient motion between image acquisition.

Modulation transfer function (MTF) Mathematical procedure for measuring spatial and contrast resolution.

Monoenergetic One energy. x- or γ-rays having a single energy.

Multiplanar reformation Use of the original transverse images to produce image data in another body plane.

Nano- Prefix that divides a basic unit by 1 billion or 10^{-9}.

Newton Unit of force in the SI system. One newton corresponds to approximately ¼ lb.

Node One of the stations or terminals of a computer network.

Noise a. Grainy or uneven appearance of an image caused by an insufficient number of primary x-rays. b. Uniform signal produced by scattered x-rays. c. Speckled appearance of the CT image caused by insufficient x-rays reaching the detectors.

Nonequilibrium Phase Phase of contrast enhancement that follows the bolus phase. It is characterized by a difference of 10 to 30 Hounsfield Units between the aorta and the inferior vena cava.

Nuclear Regulatory Commission (NRC) Federal agency that regulates the production and use of radioactive material.

Oblique Plane Imaginary plane that is slanted and lies at an angle to one of the three standard planes.

Occupational exposure Radiation exposure received by radiation workers.

Off-focus radiation X-rays emitted from parts of an anode other than the focal spot.

Optical Disk Newest type of data storage device. Consists of a disk that resembles a compact disk used to record music.

Osmolality Structural property of a liquid regarding the number of particles in solution compared to water.

Overscan Scan produced from 360° of tube travel plus approximately the width of the field of view.

Partial Scan Scans produced from a tube arc of less than 360°. Typically acquired from 180 degrees of tube travel, plus the degree of arc from the fan angle. Also called half-scan.

Partial Volume Effect Distortion of the signal intensity from an object because it extends partially into an adjacent slice thickness. Process in CT by which different tissues are averaged in a single pixel. Also known as volume averaging.

Particulate radiation As distinct from x- and γ-rays, examples are α particles, electrons, neutrons, and protons.

Penetrability Ability of x-rays to penetrate tissue. Range in tissue. X-ray quality.

Penetrometer Aluminum step wedge.

Personnel monitoring Determination of occupational radiation exposure by means of dosimetry.

Phantom Device that simulates some parameters of the human body for evaluating imager performance.

Photoconductor Material that conducts electrons when illuminated.

Photodiode Solid-state device that converts light into an electric current.

Photoelectric effect Interaction between an x-ray and an atom in which the x-ray ceases to exist and an electron is ejected from its inner shell. Absorption of an x-ray by ionization.

Photoelectron Electron ejected during the process of photoelectric effect.

Photomultiplier tube Electron tube that converts visible light into an electrical signal.

Photon Smallest quantity of electromagnetic radiation; an x-ray, gamma ray, or light. Electromagnetic radiation that has neither mass nor electric charge but interacts with matter as though it is a particle.

Photostimulation Emission of visible light following excitation by laser light.

Pico- Prefix that divides a basic unit by 1 trillion or 10^{-12}.

Pitch Table speed divided by slice thickness in spiral CT.

Pixel Picture Element of a digital image. Each pixel is assigned a CT number for image display purposes. Cell of a digital image matrix.

Polyenergetic Radiation such as x-rays having many energies. Refers to a spectrum of energies.

Potential difference Difference in voltage between two points in a circuit.

Power Time-rate at which work is done. The rate of change in energy with time. Expressed in watts (W). $1 \text{ W} = 1 \text{ J/s}$.

Primary beam (See Primary radiation.)

Primary protective barrier Barrier in the line of a primary radiation beam.

Primary radiation X-rays that emerge from an x-ray tube target confined by collimation to the area of anatomical interest; x-rays used to form an image.

Protective apparel Items of clothing (i.e., aprons, gloves) that attenuate x-rays to provide radiation protection.

Protective barrier Barrier of radiation-absorbing material used to reduce radiation exposure.

Protective housing Lead-lined metal container in which an x-ray tube is positioned. Must reduce leakage radiation to 100mR/m at 1m.

Protocol Procedure to be used when performing a quality control measurement or related operation.

Quality assurance All planned and systematic actions necessary to provide adequate confidence that a facility, system, or administrative component will perform a safe and satisfactory service to a patient. Includes scheduling, preparation, and promptness in the examination or treatment and reporting the results, as well as quality control.

Quality control Included in quality assurance, comprises all actions necessary to control and verify the performance of equipment.

Quantum detection efficiency (QDE) Relative number of x-rays that interact with a detector.

Quantum theory Physics of electromagnetic radiation and of matter smaller than an atom.

Rad (radiation absorbed dose) Special unit absorbed dose. $1 \text{ rad} = 100 \text{ erg/g} = 0.01 \text{ Gy}$.

Radiation Energy emitted and transferred through matter.

Radiation (thermal) Transfer of heat by emission of infrared electromagnetic radiation.

Radiation biology Branch of biology concerned with the effects of ionizing radiation on living systems.

Radiation quality Relative penetrability of an x-ray beam determined by its average energy; usually measured by HVL or kVp.

Radiation quantity Intensity of radiation; usually measured in mR or in Gy_a air kerma.

Radiation safety officer (RSO) Qualified individual designated by an institution to ensure that accepted guidelines for radiation protection are followed.

Radiation standards Recommendations, rules, and regulations regarding permissible concentrations, safe handling techniques, transportation, and control of radioactive material.

Radiation survey instruments Area monitoring devices that detect and/or measure radiation.

Radiation weighting factor (W_R) Factor used for radiation protection purposes that accounts for differences in biological effectiveness between different radiations. Formerly called **quality factor** (Q).

Radiological Society of North America (RSNA) Scientific society of radiologists and medical physicists.

Radiology Branch of medicine dealing with diagnostic and therapeutic applications of radiation in imaging or treatment.

Radiolucent Tissue or material that transmits x-rays and appears dark on a radiograph; transparent to x-rays.

Radiopaque Tissue or material that absorbs x-rays and appears bright on a radiograph.

Raw Data All measurements obtained from the detector array. Also called **scan data**.

Ray Sum Measurement by the detector of how much the x-ray beam has been attenuated.

Reconstruction Creating an image from data.

Reconstruction time Time after completion of examination for the computer to present a digital image.

Reformat Use of image data to create a view in a different body plane.

Region of Interest (ROI) Area of anatomy on a reconstructed digital CT image that may be circular, square, elliptic, rectangular, or custom-drawn by the operator. Defining an ROI is the first step in a number of image display and measurement functions.

Rem (radiation equivalent man) Special unit for dose equivalent and effective dose. Replaced by the sievert (Sv) in the SI system. $1 \text{ rem} = 0.01 \text{ Sv}$.

Remnant radiation All x-rays that pass through a patient and interact with the image receptor.

Resolution Measure of the ability to image objects with fidelity.

Roentgen (R) Unit of exposure to x and y radiation. 1 R = 2.58 × 10^{-4} C/kg.

Sagittal Plane Imaginary plane parallel to the long axis that divides the body into right and left sections.

Scalar Quantity or measurement that has only magnitude, as opposed to vector.

Scan Motion of x-ray tube and detector array required to collect data for reconstructing CT image.

Scan Data All measurements obtained from the detector array. Also called raw data.

Scanned Field of View Area within the gantry for which raw data are acquired. Also called calibration field of view.

Scan Parameters Factors that are controlled by the operator and affect the quality of the CT image. These factors include milliampere, kilovolt-peak, scan time, slice thickness, field of view and algorithm.

Scanned projection radiography Generalized method of making a digital radiograph; used in CT for precision localization.

Scanner Device to produce an axial or transverse sectional image. Preferred terminology is **imager**.

Scanner Generation Identified by the configuration of the x-ray tube to the detector.

Scattered radiation X-rays that change direction after an interaction with matter; Classical and Compton scattering.

Scout image Image used to localize specific body part.

Secondary protective barrier Barrier that affords protection from secondary radiation.

Secondary radiation Leakage and scatter radiation.

Semiconductor Material that can serve both as a conductor and as an insulator of electricity.

Sensitivity Ability of an image receptor to respond to x-rays; minimum signal that can be detected.

Shadow Shield Shield of radiopaque material suspended from a radiographic beam-defining system to cast a shadow in the primary beam over the patient.

Shielding Material that absorbs ionizing radiation and thus protects personnel and public.

Sievert (Sv) Special name for the SI unit of dose equivalent and effective dose. 1 Sv = 1J/kg = 100 rem.

Signal Information content of variation in current or voltage in a receiver.

Signal-to-noise-ratio (SNR) Sensitivity of a detector in recognizing a signal in the presence of background noise.

Sinusoidal Simple motion; a sine wave.

Slice Cross-sectional thickness of body part that is scanned for generating CT image.

Slice Misregistration Problem caused when the patient breathes inconsistently between images. It can result in missing areas of anatomy in the CT study.

Slip-Ring Mechanism in some CT scanners that allows the x-ray tube to rotate continually in the same direction.

SOD Source-to-object distance.

Software Computer programs that control CT imagers.

Source Collimator Device that resembles small shutters with an opening that adjust according to the operator's selection of slice thickness.

Source-to-skin distance (SSD) Distance between an x-ray tube target and the skin of a patient.

Space charge Electron cloud near the filament.

Spatial frequency Method of expressing size. A measure of the changes in tissue attenuation characteristics. Abrupt changes in tissue (e.g., at the bone-lung interface) have high spatial frequency, and gradual changes (e.g., at the liver-spleen interface) have low spatial frequency. Expressed in line pair per millimeter (1 p/mm).

Spatial resolution Ability to image anatomical structures or small objects of high contrast. High-contrast resolution.

Spectrum Graphic representation of the range over which a quantity extends.

Spiral CT Continually rotating x-ray tube with constant x-ray output and uninterrupted table movement. Also called helical, volumetric, or continuous acquisition scanning.

SSD Source-to-skin distance.

Standard Material or substance whose properties are believed to be known with sufficient accuracy to permit its use in evaluating the same properties of other materials.

Stochastic effects Probability or frequency of the biological response to radiation as a function of radiation dose. Disease incidence increases proportionately with dose, and there is no dose threshold.

Structure mottle Distribution of phosphor crystals in an intensifying screen.

Subtraction A method of removing overlying anatomy to better view small anatomy such as vessels in angiography.

Target Region of the anode struck by electrons emitted by the filament; the source of x-radiation.

Technique factors kVp and mAs as selected for a given radiation examination.

Tenth-value layer (TVL) Thickness of absorber necessary to reduce an x-ray beam to one-tenth its original intensity. 1 TVL = 3.3 HVL.

Test object Passive device of geometric shapes designed to evaluate performance of CT imagers. (See **Phantom**.)

Thermal energy Energy of molecular motion; heat; infrared radiation.

Thermionic emission Emission of electrons from a heated surface.

Thermoluminescent dosimeter (TLD) Personnel monitoring device that most often contains a crystalline form (chips or powder) of lithium fluoride as its sensing material.

Thompson scattering (See **Classical scattering**.)

Tissue weighting factor (W_T) Proportion of the risk of stochastic effects resulting from irradiation of the whole body when only an organ or tissue is irradiated.

Tomogram X-ray image of a coronal, sagittal, transverse, or oblique section through the body.

Total filtration Inherent filtration plus added filtration.

Transaxial Across the body; transverse.

Transformer Electrical device operating on the principle of mutual induction to change the magnitude of current and voltage.

Transverse Across the body; transaxial.

Tungsten Metal element that is the principal component of the cathode and the anode.

Uncontrolled area Area in which members of the general public may be found.

Use factor (U) Proportional amount of time during which an x-ray beam is energized and directed toward a particular barrier.

Useful beam (See **Primary radiation**.)

Vector Quantity or measurement that has magnitude and direction.

View Complete set of ray sums. Many views are used to produce a single CT image.

Volume Averaging When a voxel contains different tissue, the tissues are averaged and produce a CT number that represents neither. Also called partial volume effect.

Voxel Volume element—basic element that defines volume of tissue that each pixel represents in reconstructed image.

Window level Location on a CT number scale where the levels of grays are assigned; regulates the optical density of the displayed image; the center CT value of the window width.

Window width The number of gray levels or CT numbers assigned to an image; regulates the contrast of the displayed image; the range of Hounsfield units that will be represented on a particular image.

Work Product of the force on an object and the distance over which the force acts. Expressed in joules (J). W = Fd.

Workload (W) Product of the maximum milliamperage (mA) and the number of x-ray examinations performed per week. Expressed in mAmin/wk.

X-ray high-voltage generator Device that transforms electric energy from the potential supplied to that required to produce x-rays.

X-ray imager X-ray system designed for radiography, tomography, or fluoroscopy.

X-rays High energy penetrating ionizing electromagnetic radiation having a wavelength much shorter than that of visible light.

Z Axis Plane that correlates to the slice thickness, or position, of a CT slice; the long axis of a CT patient.

Additional Resources

American Association of Physicists in Medicine
One Physics Ellipse
College Park, MD 20740
Phone: 301-209-3350
Fax: 301-209-0862
Web: *www.aapm.org*

American College of Medical Physics
11250 Roger Bacon Drive
Reston, VA 22091-5202
Phone: 703-481-5001
Fax: 703-435-4390
Web: *www.acmp.org*

American College of Radiology (ACR)
11250 Roger Bacon Drive
Reston, VA 22091-5202
Phone: 703-481-5001
Fax: 703-435-4390
Web: *www.acr.org.*

American Registry of Radiologic Technologists (AART)
1255 Northland Dr.
St. Paul, MN 55120-1155
Phone: 612-687-0048
Fax: 612-687-0449

American Roentgen Ray Society
1891 Preston White Dr.
Reston, VA 22091
Phone: 703-648-8992
Fax: 703-264-8863
Toll Free: 800-439-2777
Web: *www.arrs.org*

Bushberg JT, Seibert JA, Leidholdt EMJr, Boone JM
The Essential Physics of Medical Imaging
Williams & Wilkins
Baltimore, 1994

Bushong SC
Radiologic Science for Technologists—Physics, Biology and Protection, 6th ed. Mosby—Year Book
St. Louis, 1997

Carlton RR, Adler AM
Principles of Radiographic Imaging—An Art and a Science
Delmar Publishers
Albany, NY, 1992

Educational Reviews, Inc.
6801 Cahaba Valley Rd.
Birmingham, AL 35242
Phone: 205-991-5188
Fax: 205-995-1926
Toll Free: 800-633-4743

Educational Symposia, Inc.
1527 Dale Mabry hwy.
Tampa, FL 33629-5808
Phone: 813-254-9773
Fax: 813-254-9773
Toll Free: 800-338-5901
Web: www.edusymp.com

Euclid Seeram
Computed Tomography—Physical Principles' Clinical Applications & Quality Control
W.B. Saunders Company
Philadelphia, 1994

GE Medical Systems
PO Box 414 (W-412)
Milwaukee, WI 53201
Fax: 414-544-3384
Toll Free: 800-643-6439
Web: *www.ge.com*

Hendee WR, Ritenour ER
Medical Imaging Physics, 3rd ed. Mosby—Year Book
St. Louis, 1992

Hitachi Medical Corp of America
660 White Plains Rd.
Tarrytown, NY 10591
Phone: 914-524-9711
Fax: 914-524-9716
Toll Free: 800-852-2080
Web: *www.hitachimed.com*

Huda W, Slone RM
Review of Radiologic Physics
Williams & Wilkins
Baltimore, 1995

Institute for Advanced Medical Education
15 Elm Pl
Rye, NY 10580
Phone: 914-921-5700
Fax: 914-921-6048

Lois E. Romans, R.T.
Introduction to Computed Tomography
Williams & Wilkins, 1995

Medical Technology Management Institute (MTMI)
9722 W Watertown Plank Rd.
P.O. Box 26337
Milwaukee, WI 53226-0337
Phone: 414-774-2233
Fax: 414-774-8498
Toll Free: 800-765-6864

Philips Medical Systems
North America Company
710 Bridgeport Avenue
Shelton, Connecticut 06484
Web: *www.medical.philips.com*

Picker International, Inc.
595 Miner Road
Cleveland, Ohio 44143
Phone: 216-473-3000
Fax: 216-473-2413
Web: *www.picker.com*

Rosenbusch G, Oudkerk M, Ammann E
**Radiology in Medical Diagnostics—Evolution of X-ray
    Applications 1895–1995**
Blackwell Science
London, 1995

RSNA Membership Publications
2021 Spring Rd., Suite 600
Oakbrook, IL 60521
Phone: 630-571-2670
Fax: 630-571-7837
Web: *www.rsna.org*

Siemens Medical Systems, Inc.
186 Wood Avenue
South Iselin, NJ 08880-0401
Phone: 732-321-4500
Fax: 732-494-2250
Web: *www.siemens.vents.com*

Sprawls Perry, Jr.
Physical Principles of Medical Imaging
Aspen Publishers
Gaithersburg, MD, 1993

Thompson MA, Hattaway MP, Hall JD, Dowd SB
Principles of Imaging Science and Protection
WB Saunders, Philadelphia, 1994

Answers to Practice Questions

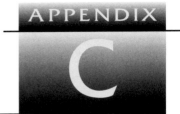

Chapter 1

1. c
2. b
3. c
4. e
5. b
6. b
7. c
8. b
9. b
10. e
11. d
12. c
13. d
14. b
15. d
16. a
17. b
18. b
19. b
20. d
21. b
22. c
23. c
24. c
25. a
26. b
27. a

Chapter 2

1. c
2. d
3. d
4. d
5. c
6. c
7. c
8. e
9. e
10. e
11. e
12. e
13. c
14. e
15. e
16. e
17. c
18. c
19. c
20. d
21. c
22. e
23. d
24. e
25. c
26. d
27. d
28. e
29. d
30. c
31. e
32. c
33. b
34. d
35. a
36. d
37. c
38. e
39. d
40. d
41. d
42. e
43. b
44. c
45. b
46. d
47. d
48. c
49. c
50. a
51. d
52. d
53. b

Chapter 3

1. b
2. a
3. b
4. b
5. c
6. d
7. b
8. e
9. d
10. c
11. b
12. c
13. d
14. a
15. c
16. e
17. b
18. a
19. c
20. d
21. d
22. e
23. c
24. c
25. b
26. d
27. e
28. b
29. a
30. d
31. d
32. d
33. a
34. b
35. b
36. b
37. e
38. d
39. b
40. e
41. d

42. d
43. a
44. d
45. d
46. d
47. b
48. a
49. e
50. b
51. e
52. d
53. b
54. a
55. c
56. e
57. e
58. e
59. a
60. b
61. c
62. d
63. b
64. a
65. d
66. b
67. e
68. c
69. a
70. e
71. b
72. e
73. a
74. d
75. d
76. b
77. b
78. b
79. c
80. d
81. e
82. c
83. a
84. b
85. d
86. b
87. c
88. b
89. d
90. b
91. a
92. c
93. d
94. b
95. e
96. e

97. c
98. d
99. b
100. e
101. c

Chapter 4
1. a
2. b
3. c
4. e
5. b
6. e
7. d
8. e
9. a
10. d
11. a
12. c
13. d
14. e
15. e
16. b
17. e
18. d
19. d
20. a
21. e
22. a
23. c
24. e
25. b
26. a
27. a
28. b
29. d
30. a
31. d
32. c
33. b
34. c
35. a
36. b
37. d
38. b
39. b
40. e
41. e
42. e
43. e
44. b
45. e
46. a
47. a

48. e
49. e
50. b
51. d
52. c
53. e
54. a
55. e
56. e
57. d
58. c
59. a
60. e
61. d
62. e
63. b
64. c
65. a
66. a
67. c
68. a
69. a
70. c
71. a
72. b
73. a
74. a
75. b
76. a
77. d
78. e
79. c
80. d
81. c
82. c
83. a
84. a
85. b
86. e
87. b
88. a
89. d
90. a
91. e
92. b
93. a
94. d
95. a
96. b
97. a
98. b
99. e
100. e
101. a
102. d

Chapter 5
1. a
2. e
3. e
4. e
5. c
6. b
7. d
8. a
9. a
10. c
11. a
12. e
13. a
14. c
15. d
16. c
17. b
18. e
19. b
20. e
21. d
22. c
23. d
24. e
25. b
26. b
27. b
28. e
29. c
30. c
31. d
32. b
33. b
34. e
35. b
36. c
37. e
38. c
39. d
40. d
41. b
42. b
43. e
44. d
45. d
46. b
47. d
48. c
49. e
50. e
51. c
52. e
53. e
54. d

55. a
56. a
57. c
58. d
59. a
60. c
61. c
62. b
63. e
64. a
65. c
66. c
67. d
68. c
69. d
70. e
71. a
72. b
73. b
74. a

Chapter 6
1. a
2. d
3. b
4. d
5. c
6. b
7. c
8. a
9. b
10. e
11. e
12. a
13. a
14. e

Chapter 7
1. e
2. b
3. b
4. e
5. e
6. c
7. e
8. e
9. b
10. e
11. c
12. a
13. e
14. e

15. b
16. b
17. b
18. a
19. a
20. d
21. b
22. e
23. b
24. e
25. b
26. e
27. a
28. b
29. a
30. a
31. d
32. a
33. a
34. e
35. c
36. c
37. c
38. a
39. a
40. a
41. b
42. d
43. e
44. b
45. b
46. a
47. d
48. e
49. a
50. a
51. b
52. b
53. b
54. d
55. c
56. c
57. a
58. d
59. b
60. b
61. b
62. d
63. d
64. e
65. a
66. a
67. b
68. c
69. a

70. d
71. c
72. c
73. b
74. b
75. a
76. e
77. d

Chapter 8
1. b
2. a
3. e
4. c
5. a
6. e
7. a
8. e
9. d
10. a
11. d
12. b
13. e
14. c
15. a
16. e
17. a

18. a
19. c
20. c

Chapter 9
1. a
2. d
3. b
4. e
5. e
6. a
7. b
8. a
9. a
10. b
11. e
12. b
13. a
14. a
15. a
16. a
17. b
18. a
19. a
20. d
21. a
22. d

23. a
24. d

Chapter 10
1. c
2. b
3. b
4. a
5. d
6. c
7. a
8. c
9. a
10. e
11. c
12. a
13. b
14. a
15. d
16. e
17. c
18. a
19. e
20. a
21. a
22. b
23. c